Multiple Choice Questions for Haematology and Core Medical Trainees

T0355652

This title is also available as an e-book. For more details, please see
www.wiley.com/buy/9781119210528
or scan this QR code:

Multiple Choice Questions for Haematology and Core Medical Trainees

Barbara J. Bain

MB BS, FRACP, FRCPath
Professor in Diagnostic Haematology,
Imperial College London and Honorary Consultant Haematologist,
St Mary's Hospital, Praed Street, London.

WILEY Blackwell

This edition first published 2016 © 2016 by John Wiley & Sons Ltd.

Registered office:
John Wiley & Sons, Ltd, The Atrium, Southern Gate, Chichester, West Sussex, PO19 8SQ, UK

Editorial offices:
9600 Garsington Road, Oxford, OX4 2DQ, UK
1606 Golden Aspen Drive, Suites 103 and 104, Ames, Iowa 50010, USA

For details of our global editorial offices, for customer services and for information about how to apply for permission to reuse the copyright material in this book please see our website at www.wiley.com/wiley-blackwell

Library of Congress Cataloging-in-Publication Data

Names: Bain, Barbara J., author.
Title: Multiple choice questions for haematology and core medical trainees / Barbara J. Bain.
Description: Chichester, West Sussex, UK ; Ames, Iowa : John Wiley & Sons,
    Inc., [2016] | Includes bibliographical references and index.
Identifiers: LCCN 2015044915 (print) | LCCN 2015047076 (ebook) |
    ISBN 9781119210528 (pbk.) | ISBN 9781119210559 (pdf) | ISBN 9781119210535 (epub)
Subjects: | MESH: Hematologic Diseases—Examination Questions. | Blood
    Physiological Phenomena—Examination Questions.
Classification: LCC RC633 (print) | LCC RC633 (ebook) | NLM WH 18.2 |
    DDC 616.1/50076—dc23
LC record available at http://lccn.loc.gov/2015044915

A catalogue record for this book is available from the British Library.

Wiley also publishes its books in a variety of electronic formats. Some content that appears in print may not be available in electronic books.

Set in 9/11.5pt MeridienLTStd-Roman by Thomson Digital, Noida, India

1   2016

Contents

Preface   vii

Normal Ranges and Abbreviations   ix

Section 1: Single Best Answers
           Questions 1–50   1

Section 2: Single Best Answers
           Questions 51–120   29

Section 3: Extended Matching Questions 1–30   67

Section 4: Single Best Answers
           Answers to Questions 1–120 with Feedback   101

Section 5: Extended Matching Questions
           Answers and Feedback   155

Index   187

Preface

This book has been written to help haematology trainees preparing for the part 1 examination of the Royal College of Pathologists. It will also be of use to core medical trainees preparing for the examinations of the Royal College of Physicians and the Royal Australasian College of Physicians and to haematology and general medicine trainees in other countries where methods of examination are similar. There is a considerable paediatric content so the book will also be useful to those preparing for examination of the Royal College of Paediatrics and Child Health. The two formats that are most used by these Royal Colleges have been used, Single Best Answer and Extended Matching Question. Detailed feedback and, when appropriate, relevant references are given for each question so that those who select the wrong answer will understand why another answer is preferred. Because of the detailed feedback and because some of the questions are quite searching, the book is an educational tool as well as a way to prepare for examinations. It will thus be of value also to advanced trainees including those preparing for the part 2 RCPath examination. Since the book incorporates much recent knowledge it may well also be of use to consultant haematologists wanting to update themselves as well as to those who are involved in training and examining.

Barbara J. Bain, 2016

Normal Ranges and Abbreviations

Core abbreviations and normal ranges

Standard abbreviations (not defined in text) and normal ranges for the full blood count (FBC) in Caucasian adults are shown in this table. Normal ranges for children and for other tests are given in relation to the individual cases when necessary.

	Males	Females	Units
White blood cell count (WBC)	3.7–7.9	3.9–11.1	× 10^9/l
Red blood cell count (RBC)	4.32–5.66	3.88–4.99	× 10^{12}/l
Haemoglobin concentration (Hb)	133–167	118–148	g/l
Haematocrit (Hct)	0.39–0.50	0.36–0.44	l/l
Mean cell volume (MCV)	82–98		fl
Mean cell haemoglobin (MCH)	27.3–32.6		pg
Mean cell haemoglobin concentration (MCHC)	316–349		g/l
Neutrophils	1.7–6.1	1.7–7.5	× 10^9/l
Lymphocytes	1.0–3.2		× 10^9/l
Monocytes	0.2–0.6		× 10^9/l
Eosinophils	0.03–0.06		× 10^9/l
Basophils	0.02–0.29		× 10^9/l
Platelets	143–332	169–358	× 10^9/l

Other abbreviations

aHUS	atypical haemolytic uraemic syndrome
ABVD	doxorubicin, bleomycin, vinblastine, dacarbazine
ADAMTS13	a disintegrin and metalloproteinase with a thrombospondin type 1 motif, member 13
AIDS	acquired immune deficiency syndrome
ALL	acute lymphoblastic leukaemia
AML	acute myeloid leukaemia
APTT	activated partial thromboplastin time
ATLL	adult T-cell leukaemia/lymphoma
BEACOPP	bleomycin, etoposide, doxorubicin, cyclophosphamide, vincristine, procarbazine, prednisone
C	complement
CD	cluster of differentiation
CHOP	cyclophosphamide, doxorubicin, vincristine, prednisolone
CLL	chronic lymphocytic leukaemia
CT	computed tomography
DNA	deoxyribonucleic acid
DVT	deep vein thrombosis
ESR	erythrocyte sedimentation rate
G6PD	glucose-6-phosphate dehydrogenase
HIT	heparin-induced thrombocytopenia
HIV	human immunodeficiency virus
HPLC	high performance liquid chromatography
Ig	immunoglobulin
INR	international normalised ratio
LDH	lactate dehydrogenase
MALT	mucosa-associated lymphoid tissue
MRI	magnetic resonance imaging
NK	natural killer
NRBC	nucleated red blood cells
PET	positron emission tomography
PNH	paroxysmal nocturnal haemoglobinuria
PT	prothrombin time
R-CHOP	rituximab + CHOP
RDW	red cell distribution width
RiCoF	ristocetin co-factor
RNA	ribonucleic acid
SLE	systemic lupus erythematosus
TdT	terminal deoxynucleotidyl transferase
TTP	thrombotic thrombocytopenic purpura
VWF	von Willebrand factor

Section 1:
Single Best Answers
Questions 1–50

This section comprises 50 Single Best Answer (SBA) questions. They are divided into questions 1–31, which are more relevant to the part 1 MRCP examination and questions 32–50, which are more relevant to the part 2 MRCP examination. Although having a general medical slant, these questions are also appropriate for haematology specialist trainees. Normal ranges are given in parentheses. Answers and feedback will be found on pages 101–123.

Multiple Choice Questions for Haematology and Core Medical Trainees, First Edition.
Barbara J. Bain.
© 2016 John Wiley & Sons, Ltd. Published 2016 by John Wiley & Sons, Ltd.

MRCP part 1 level

SBA 1

A 69-year-old Afro-Caribbean woman is referred to rheumatology out-patients because of painful joints and morning stiffness. She is found to have a minor degree of lymphadenopathy and her spleen is tipped on inspiration. An FBC shows WBC 98×10^9/l, Hb 83 g/l, platelet count 221×10^9/l, neutrophils 7.2×10^9/l and lymphocytes 91×10^9/l. Her blood film shows mature small lymphocytes with scanty cytoplasm, round nuclei and coarsely clumped chromatin. Smear cells are present. Rheumatoid factor is detected and her erythrocyte sedimentation rate (ESR) is 54 mm in 1 h (<20).

The most likely diagnosis is:

a Adult T-cell leukaemia/lymphoma
b Chronic lymphocytic leukaemia
c Follicular lymphoma in leukaemic phase
d Mantle cell lymphoma
e Reactive lymphocytosis

SBA 2

A 69-year-old man who has received repeated courses of chemotherapy and chemo-immunotherapy for refractory mantle cell lymphoma presents with the gradual onset of cognitive impairment, dysphasia and dyspraxia. On lumbar puncture, pressure is normal, there is a slight increase in protein concentration, cell count is not increased and glucose is normal. Magnetic resonance imaging (MRI) of the brain shows multiple high intensity signals on T2-weighted and FLAIR sequences affecting mainly the white matter.

The most likely organism implicated is:

a BK virus
b Herpes simplex
c JC virus
d *Treponema pallidum*
e Varicella-zoster virus

SBA 3

A 49-year-old woman is admitted to the intensive care ward with septic shock. Her FBC shows WBC $18 \times 10^9/l$, Hb 83 g/l, platelet count $150 \times 10^9/l$, neutrophils $17.2 \times 10^9/l$ and lymphocytes $0.5 \times 10^9/l$. Her blood film shows toxic granulation and left shift.

The appropriate haemoglobin threshold for blood transfusion in this patient would be:

a 60 g/l
b 70 g/l
c 80 g/l
d 90 g/l
e 100 g/l

SBA 4

A 23-year-old woman is hospitalised with severe anorexia nervosa. Her FBC shows WBC $3.5 \times 10^9/l$, neutrophil count $1.1 \times 10^9/l$, Hb 100 g/l, MCV 104 fl and platelet count $70 \times 10^9/l$. Blood film shows occasional acanthocytes. Neutrophils show normal segmentation. Her prothrombin time (PT) is slightly increased.

The most likely diagnosis is:

a Aplastic anaemia
b Folic acid deficiency
c Haematological features of anorexia nervosa
d Hepatic steatosis
e Vitamin B_{12} deficiency

SBA 5

A 60-year-old Cypriot woman is referred back to rheumatology outpatients as she has suffered a flare of her rheumatoid arthritis. Her FBC shows WBC $12.0 \times 10^9/l$, RBC $3.62 \times 10^{12}/l$, Hb 83 g/l, Hct 0.27 l/l, MCV 74 fl, MCHC 310 g/l, platelet count $441 \times 10^9/l$ and neutrophils $9.2 \times 10^9/l$. Her blood film shows increased rouleaux formation and the ESR is 65 mm in 1 h (<20). Serum ferritin is 47 µg/l (14–200), serum iron is 6 µmol/l (11–28) and total iron binding capacity 65 µmol/l (45–75).

The most likely explanation of the microcytic anaemia is:

a α thalassaemia trait
b Anaemia of chronic disease
c Anaemia of chronic disease plus iron deficiency
d β thalassaemia trait
e Iron deficiency

SBA 6

A 60-year-old Caucasian man presents with a history of fatigue, nausea, abdominal discomfort, altered bowel function, insomnia, anxiety and altered taste. He is a self-employed painter and decorator with a past history of a coronary artery bypass and is taking atorvastatin. His FBC shows WBC $7.8 \times 10^9/l$, Hb 105 g/l, Hct 0.30 l/l, MCV 79 fl, MCH 27.6 pg, MCHC 350 g/l, red cell distribution width (RDW) 15% (9.5–15.5), platelet count $403 \times 10^9/l$ and reticulocyte count $120 \times 10^9/l$. His blood film shows anisocytosis, polychromasia, basophilic stippling and occasional nucleated red blood cells and myelocytes. A bone marrow aspirate shows dyserythropoiesis with abnormal sideroblasts including 3% ring sideroblasts.

The most likely diagnosis is:

a Lead poisoning
b Myelodysplastic syndrome (refractory anaemia)
c Myelodysplastic syndrome (refractory anaemia with ring sideroblasts)
d Pyrimidine 5′ nucleotidase deficiency
e Zinc deficiency

SBA 7

A 57-year-old man with a history of hypercholesterolaemia, heart failure and atrial fibrillation is on warfarin with a satisfactory international normalised ratio (INR). He presents with the sudden onset of marked swelling of the left leg and thigh with pain in his foot and calf. Within a short period of time, the distal foot become purplish blue and cold with no palpable pulses in the leg.

The most likely diagnosis is:

a Embolisation from the left atrium
b Femoral artery thrombosis
c Plegmasia alba dolens
d Plegmasia caerulea dolens
e Worsening heart failure

SBA 8

A 32-year-old woman with a history of irritable bowel syndrome is found to have iron deficiency anaemia and a serum folate of 1 µg/l (2–11). Her serum vitamin B_{12} is normal. Her diet is assessed as nutritionally adequate, although she says she has to 'watch what she eats'.

The test you would do next is:

a Antibodies to deamidated gliadin peptide
b Antiendomysial antibodies
c Antiendomysial antibodies, making sure that the patient is first on a gluten-free diet
d Duodenal biopsy
e Ig (immunoglobulin) A anti-tissue transglutaminase antibodies

SBA 9

A 23-year-old African man who presents with an epileptiform convulsion and fever is found to have a microangiopathic haemolytic anaemia, thrombocytopenia and acute kidney injury.

The micro-organism you would test for is:

a *Escherichia coli* O104:H4
b *Escherichia coli* O157:H7
c Hepatitis B
d Human herpesvirus 8
e Human immunodeficiency virus

SBA 10

An 18-year-old medical student is permitted to perform an unsupervised venepuncture on a febrile Indian patient and suffers a needle prick injury. He is anxious that he may have contracted human immunodeficiency virus (HIV) infection.

Assuming that the patient is infected, transmission is most likely for:

a Dengue fever
b Hepatitis B
c Hepatitis C
d Human immunodeficiency virus (HIV)
e Leishmaniasis

SBA 11

A 39-year-old woman presents with haemoptysis and is found to have a pulmonary arteriovenous malformation. She is also noted to be pale and to have telangiectasia of the lips and tongue. There are no other abnormal physical findings. A full blood count shows WBC 7.2 × 10⁹/l, RBC 3.10 × 10¹²/l, Hb 70 g/l, Hct 0.23 l/l, MCV 75.6 fl, MCH 23.8 pg, MCHC 315 g/l and platelet count 221 × 10⁹/l.

The most likely underlying diagnosis is:

a Acquired von Willebrand disease
b Advanced liver disease
c CREST variant of scleroderma (calcinosis, Raynaud phenomenon, (o) esophageal dysmotility, sclerodactyly, telangiectasia)
d Hereditary haemorrhagic telangiectasia
e Heyde syndrome

SBA 12

A 29-year-old man suffered a road traffic accident in West Africa and required a splenectomy. A few weeks after his return to the UK he presents with chills, fever, myalgia and vomiting. He is found to be hypotensive with no localising signs. His FBC shows WBC 18 × 10⁹/l, Hb 177 g/l, platelet count 98 × 10⁹/l, neutrophils 17.2 × 10⁹/l and lymphocytes 0.6 × 10⁹/l. His blood film shows toxic granulation and left shift. No malaria parasites are seen on thick film examination. A coagulation screen shows a prolonged activated partial thromboplastin time (APTT) and increased D dimers.

The lost likely cause of the fever is infection by:

a *Capnocytophaga canimorsus*
b *Haemophilus influenza* type b
c *Neisseria meningitidis*
d *Plasmodium falciparum*
e *Streptococcus pneumonia*

SBA 13

A 52-year-old man with poor prognosis acute myeloid leukaemia achieves a complete remission with daunorubicin and cytarabine. He then receives an allogeneic haemopoietic stem cell transplant from a matched unrelated donor after conditioning with busulphan and cyclophosphamide. He receives methotrexate and tacrolimus for graft-versus-host disease prophylaxis. A week after transplantation he complains of abdominal pain and is found to have a tender liver, weight gain, oedema and ascites. His bilirubin has risen to 35 µmol/l (<17) and alanine aminotransferase is twice the upper limit of normal. Creatinine has risen to 132 µmol/l (60–125).

The most likely diagnosis is:

a Graft-versus-host disease
b Hepatorenal syndrome
c Inferior vena cava thrombosis
d Methotrexate toxicity
e Sinusoidal obstruction syndrome

SBA 14

A 30-year-old woman is referred to medical outpatients with suspected hypothyroidism. On reviewing her clinical history it is found that she was treated abroad for Hodgkin lymphoma at the age of 16 years with mantle radiotherapy and combination chemotherapy (doxorubicin, bleomycin, vinblastine and dacarbazine).

The long term morbidity of the treatment administered to this patient includes a significantly increased rate of:

a Acute lymphoblastic and acute myeloid leukaemia
b Acute myeloid leukaemia, breast cancer, hypothyroidism and coronary artery disease
c Bladder cancer
d Breast and ovarian cancer
e Hypothyroidism

SBA 15

A 29-year-old Caucasian woman who is seen in outpatients for review of the management of her coeliac disease mentions that she has been trying to get pregnant for some time. She has previously been deficient in both folic acid and iron but her blood count is now normal

You advise her that when trying to get pregnant:

a She does not need any dietary supplements
b She should take supplementary ferrous sulphate
c She should take supplementary folic acid
d She should take supplementary pyridoxine
e She should take supplementary vitamin B_{12}

SBA 16

A 43-year-old woman presents with sudden onset of blurred vision in both eyes. She is tired and has suffered from recurrent aphthous ulcers. Ophthalmological examination shows multiple bilateral retinal haemorrhages without exudates; optic discs appeared normal. Visual acuity is reduced. FBC shows Hb 48 g/l, MCV 119 fl, WBC 6.1×10^9/l and platelet count 86×10^9/l. The blood film showed macrocytes, oval macrocytes and hypersegmented neutrophils.

The most likely cause of the retinal haemorrhages is:

a Anaemia
b Impaired platelet function
c Raised intracranial pressure
d Malignant hypertension
e Thrombocytopenia

SBA 17

A 31-year-old Caucasian woman had been known to have elevated transaminases for several years but this had not been followed up. She is teetotal. She presents in liver failure and is found to have an Hb of 74 g/l and a reticulocyte count of 270 × 10^9/l (50–100). A blood film shows irregularly contracted cells, polychromasia and nucleated red blood cells. A Heinz body preparation is positive.

The most likely diagnosis is:

a Autoimmune haemolytic anaemia
b Exposure to an exogenous oxidant
c Glucose-6-phosphate dehydrogenase (G6PD) deficiency
d Wilson's disease
e Zieve's syndrome

SBA 18

A 23-year-old Afro-Caribbean woman presents with symptoms of anaemia. She has also suffered from swollen painful joints. Her FBC shows WBC 4.5 × 10^9/l, Hb 53 g/l, MCV 93 fl, reticulocyte count 5 × 10^9/l (50–100) and platelet count 151 × 10^9/l. Her blood film shows normocytic normochromic red cells. On further testing she is found to have antinuclear activity and anti-double stranded deoxyribonucleic acid (DNA) antibodies. Creatinine is 135 µmol/l (60–125).

The likely cause of the anaemia is:

a Anaemia of chronic disease (anaemia of inflammation)
b Autoimmune haemolytic anaemia
c Chronic kidney injury
d Megaloblastic anaemia
e Pure red cell aplasia

SBA 19

An 8-year-old boy suffers an upper respiratory tract infection following which he develops abdominal pain and palpable purpura of his buttocks and shins. There are also small numbers of petechiae. His mother reports that he has passed red urine.

The most likely explanation of the purpura is:

a Autoimmune thrombocytopenic purpura
b Cryoglobulinaemia
c Disseminated intravascular coagulation
d Henoch–Schönlein purpura
e Post-infection thrombocytopenic purpura

SBA 20

A 63-year-old woman presents with morning stiffness and bilateral neck and shoulder pain and bilateral thigh pain. She has a low grade fever and has lost weight. Her muscles are tender. Polymyalgia rheumatica is suspected and her ESR is therefore measured.

The diagnostic criterion supporting this diagnosis is:

a ESR greater than 30 mm in 1 h
b ESR greater than 40 mm in 1 h
c ESR greater than 50 mm in 1 h
d ESR greater than 60 mm in 1 h
e ESR greater than 70 mm in 1 h

SBA 21

A 33-year-old woman with systemic lupus erythematosus who has developed livedo reticularis suffers an unprovoked deep vein thrombosis in her left leg. Her coagulation screen shows a PT of 16 s (12–14) and an APTT of 40 s (26–33.5).

The test most strongly indicative of your suspected diagnosis would be:

a Anti-β2 glycoprotein 1 antibodies
b Antibodies to the phosphatidylserine–prothrombin complex
c Anti-cardiolipin antibodies
d Anti-prothrombin antibodies
e Lupus anticoagulant

SBA 22

A 70-year-old man presents with symptoms of fatigue and dyspnoea. His diet is normal and his alcohol intake is low. He is on no medications. His FBC shows WBC 4.5×10^9/l, Hb 53 g/l, MCV 116 fl, reticulocyte count 20×10^9/l (50–100) and platelet count 51×10^9/l. His blood film shows marked anisocytosis and poikilocytosis with macrocytes, oval macrocytes, teardrop poikilocytes, red cell fragments, occasional keratocytes and a few hypersegmented neutrophils. Creatinine is 105 µmol/l (60–125).

The likely cause of the abnormalities found is:

a Atypical haemolytic uraemic syndrome (aHUS)
b Folic acid deficiency
c Myelodysplastic syndrome
d Thrombotic thrombocytopenic purpura (TTP)
e Vitamin B_{12} deficiency

SBA 23

A 6-month-old baby boy born to Pakistani parents presents with failure to thrive. He had been weaned on to cow's milk at an early age. He is found to have pallor and hepatosplenomegaly. His FBC shows Hb 78 g/l (99–141), MCV 65 fl (71–84) and MCH 18 pg (24–34). His blood film shows anisocytosis, poikilocytosis, hypochromia, microcytosis and some nucleated red blood cells. Serum ferritin is 25 µg/l (14–200).

The most likely diagnosis is:

a α thalassaemia
b β thalassaemia
c Congenital dyserythropoietic anaemia
d Congenital sideroblastic anaemia
e Iron deficiency anaemia

SBA 24

A 35-year-old woman has a history of hereditary spherocytosis and has an Hb of 88 g/l and a reticulocyte count of 350 × 10^9/l (50–100). She has a family history of diabetes mellitus and haemoglobin A_{1c} is therefore measured and is found to be 5%/31 mmol/mol (<6%/<42 mmol/mol).

Your interpretation of this result is:

a A valid interpretation of the haemoglobin A_{1c} is possible
b Diabetes mellitus is very unlikely
c Hereditary spherocytosis will interfere with the accuracy of the assay
d The haemoglobin A_{1c} is likely to be misleadingly elevated
e The haemoglobin A_{1c} is likely to be misleadingly reduced

SBA 25

A 70-year-old man trips on his doorstep. He develops massive bruising of his thigh and leg and heavy bleeding from a wound to the shin. He has a past medical history of myocardial infarction 20 years previously and idiopathic bile salt malabsorption, for which he is taking colestyramine. His FBC shows WBC 6.8×10^9/l, Hb 119 g/l, MCV 95 fl and platelet count 420×10^9/l. His blood film shows polychromasia. A coagulation screen shows PT >120 s (12–14), APTT 102 s (23–35), thrombin time 12 s (control 13 s) and fibrinogen concentration 3.5 g/l.

The most likely explanation of the abnormal coagulation is:

a Disseminated intravascular coagulation (DIC)
b Factor X deficiency
c Haemophilia A
d Hyperfibrinolysis
e Vitamin K malabsorption

SBA 26

You are consulted about the advisability of varicella-zoster vaccination.

You would advise vaccination in:

a An apparently healthy 70-year-old woman.
b A 70-year-old man on chemotherapy for chronic lymphocytic leukaemia
c A 40-year-old woman who has had a haemopoietic stem cell transplant for high risk acute myeloid leukaemia
d A 60-year-old man who has had a renal transplant
e A 35-year-old woman who is taking prednisolone 20 mg daily because of a flare up of systemic lupus erythematosus

SBA 27

A 25-year-old man becomes unwell 4 days after returning from a holiday in India. He is febrile with a headache, myalgia and an erythematous rash. It is noted that after his blood pressure has been taken his forearm shows petechiae. FBC shows WBC $3.3 \times 10^9/l$, Hb 170 g/l, neutrophil count $1.3 \times 10^9/l$, lymphocyte count $1.5 \times 10^9/l$ and platelet count $24 \times 10^9/l$. His blood film shows atypical lymphocytes. The neutrophils do not show toxic changes. A coagulation screen shows a slight prolongation of the PT and APTT, somewhat reduced fibrinogen concentration and increased D dimer.

The most likely diagnosis is:

a Ebola virus disease
b Dengue fever
c Malaria
d Meningococcal septicaemia
e Typhoid fever

SBA 28

An 18-year-old previously healthy student who has just returned from a trip to East Africa presents with a cough and fever, particularly at night. He also has myalgia and headache. He had noticed an itchy rash in the preceding week. He admits that he has not taken his antimalarials conscientiously. His chest X-ray shows diffuse pulmonary infiltrates. FBC shows eosinophilia.

The most likely diagnosis is:

a Eosinophilic granulomatosis with polyangiitis
b Malaria
c Miliary tuberculosis
d Schistosomiasis
e Trypanosomiasis

SBA 29

A 27-year-old man who has just returned from a holiday in Thailand presents with fever, chills and headache. His temperature is 39.4°C and his pulse rate is 100 per minute. An automated full blood count shows Hb 112 g/l, WBC 3.8×10^9/l and platelet count 95×10^9/l. There is an instrument 'flag' for atypical lymphocytes. Biochemical tests show elevated bilirubin, alanine transaminase and lactate dehydrogenase (LDH).

The physician should initiate laboratory tests for:

a Dengue fever
b Hepatitis A
c HIV infection
d Malaria
e Typhoid fever

SBA 30

A 63-year-old Greek man with rheumatoid arthritis has been taking aspirin and non-steroidal anti-inflammatory drugs. Despite this treatment he has early morning stiffness and his joints are still swollen and painful. His blood tests show an Hb of 98 g/l and an MCV of 78 fl. His serum iron and transferrin saturation are low and his serum ferritin is 115 µg/l (15–200).

The most likely diagnosis is:

a A combination of iron deficiency and anaemia of chronic disease.
b Acquired sideroblastic anaemia
c Anaemia of chronic disease
d Iron deficiency anaemia due to drug-induced intestinal blood loss
e β thalassaemia trait

SBA 31

A 23-year-old man presents with fever and dyspnoea. On examination, he appears pale and unwell, he has a number of bruises and his spleen is felt 2 cm below the left costal margin. A chest X-ray shows patchy shadowing in his lungs. His FBC shows WBC 9.2×10^9/l, Hb 89 g/l, MCV 95 fl, platelet count 41×10^9/l, neutrophils 0.7×10^9/l, lymphocytes 3.2×10^9/l, blast cells 5.2×10^9/l. Rare blast cells contain Auer rods. His neutrophils appear almost agranular and are hypolobated.

The most likely diagnosis is:

a Acute lymphoblastic leukaemia
b Acute myeloid leukaemia
c Chronic myeloid leukaemia
d High grade lymphoma
e Myelodysplastic syndrome

MRCP part 2 level

SBA 32

A 59-year-old woman presents with fatigue. Her FBC shows WBC $4.8 \times 10^9/l$, Hb 93 g/l, MCV 115 fl and platelet count $120 \times 10^9/l$. Her blood film shows macrocytes, oval macrocytes and hypersegmented neutrophils. She has a past history of Hashimoto thyroiditis.

The most specific test to confirm the diagnosis you suspect is:

a Anti-glutaminase antibodies
b Intrinsic factor antibodies
c Parietal cell antibodies
d Plasma homocysteine
e Serum vitamin B_{12}

SBA 33

A 23-year-old woman with poorly managed thalassaemia major is being evaluated for suspected iron overload. Blood tests show serum ferritin 2300 µg/l (15–200), haemoglobin A_{1c} 9.5%/80 mmol/mol (<6%, <42 mmol/mol), corrected serum calcium 1.6 mmol/l (2.15–2.55) and serum phosphate 2.1 mmol/l (0.7–1.5). A computed tomography (CT) scan of her head is carried out and shows bilateral symmetrical calcification of basal ganglia and some calcification of the cerebellum and the grey matter–white matter junction of the cerebrum.

The most likely explanation of the CT finding is:

a Calcification of sites of extramedullary erythropoiesis
b Diabetes mellitus
c Hypoparathyroidism
d Iron deposition in the brain leading to ectopic calcification
e Previous brain infarction

SBA 34

A 58-year-old woman with a previous history of breast cancer presents with tiredness. She is found to have a low grade fever and enlargement of the spleen 10 cm below the left costal margin. Her FBC shows WBC $14.8 \times 10^9/l$, Hb 74 g/l, MCV 85 fl and platelet count $500 \times 10^9/l$. Her blood film is leucoerythroblastic and shows tear drop poikilocytes.

The most likely diagnosis is:

a Essential thrombocythaemia
b Bone marrow metastases
c Chronic myeloid leukaemia
d Liver metastases causing hypersplenism
e Primary myelofibrosis

SBA 35

A 25-year-old man with known sickle cell disease has had recurrent priapism and frequent painful crises. He has often required transfusion, particularly exchange transfusion. He has also had a cholecystectomy. He develops recurrent episodes of right upper quadrant pain, hepatomegaly, fever and impaired liver function. He has extreme hyperbilirubinaemia (68% conjugated) and abnormal liver enzymes but normal serum albumin.

The most likely diagnosis is:

a Gallstone in common bile duct
b Hepatic iron overload
c Hepatic sequestration
d Sickle cell-related intrahepatic cholestasis
e Viral hepatitis

SBA 36

A 25-year-old man presents with abdominal pain and diarrhoea but without any passage of blood. He is hypertensive. His FBC shows a normal Hb and platelet count but he has a neutrophil leucocytosis with a left shift. Three days later he becomes anuric, his creatinine rises, his platelet count falls to $35 \times 10^9/l$ and schistocytes are found in his blood film. A test on stool for Shiga toxin is negative. ADAMTS13 is assayed at 75% (50–150%).

The most likely diagnosis is:

a Atypical haemolytic uraemic syndrome (aHUS)
b Disseminated intravascular coagulation (DIC)
c Haemolytic uraemic syndrome (HUS)
d Microangiopathic haemolytic anaemia due to renal cortical necrosis
e Thrombotic thrombocytopenic purpura (TTP)

SBA 37

A 56-year-old northern European man with bulky stage IV diffuse large B-cell lymphoma has recently received a first course of R-CHOP (rituximab, cyclophosphamide, doxorubicin, vincristine and prednisolone) combination chemo-immunotherapy. He develops paraesthesia and tingling in his hands and is found to have hypocalcaemia, hyperkalaemia and hyperuricaemia. Creatinine is 125 μmol/l (53–115) and potassium is 5.1 mmol/l (3.5–5.0).

In addition to vigorous hydration and careful monitoring of fluid balance and biochemical measurements, treatment indicated is:

a Allopurinol
b Haemofiltration
c Peritoneal dialysis
d Rasburicase
e Urinary alkalinisation plus allopurinol

SBA 38

A 45-year-old woman presents with a pain in her left calf, which has a circumference 1 cm greater than the right calf when measured 10 cm below the tibial tuberosity. She has a previous history of deep vein thrombosis (DVT). Her Wells' score is 0.

The most appropriate management is:

a Measure D dimer
b Perform venography
c Perform venous ultrasonography of the left leg
d Prescribe low molecular weight heparin
e Prescribe rivaroxaban

SBA 39

An 85-year-old woman with atrial fibrillation and a previous history of hypertension and hypercholesterolaemia presents with a stroke due to acute right middle cerebral artery occlusion. She is managed with thrombolysis using tissue plasminogen activator followed by warfarin with bridging enoxaparin. Three weeks later she develops fever, myalgia and painful purple feet followed by renal failure. Her INR is 4.2 and eosinophil count is $0.9 \times 10^9/l$.

The most likely diagnosis is:

a An allergic reaction to warfarin
b Antiphospholipid syndrome
c Cholesterol embolisation
d Multiple emboli resulting from atrial fibrillation
e Systemic vasculitis

SBA 40

A 45-year-old man presented with splenomegaly and generalised lymphadenopathy. Following a lymph node biopsy and a bone marrow trephine biopsy a diagnosis of stage IVA diffuse large B-cell lymphoma was made. The patient was treated with R-CHOP in standard doses. Seven days after commencing chemotherapy he complains of nausea. Biochemical investigations show a serum sodium of 123 mmol/l and potassium 3.7 mmol/l (3.5–5.0). Serum creatinine is normal. He appears euvolaemic. Serum osmolality is found to be 255 mOsm/kg (275–295) and urine osmolality 260 mOsm/kg.

The treatment indicated is:

a Administration of adrenocorticosteroids
b Fluid restriction
c Infusion of hypertonic saline
d Infusion of normal saline without supplementary potassium
e Oral tolvaptan

SBA 41

A 19-year-old West African man presents with generalised lymphadenopathy and splenomegaly. His FBC shows WBC 18×10^9/l, Hb 93 g/l and platelet count 101×10^9/l. His blood film shows circulating lymphoma cells and following further investigation a diagnosis of Burkitt lymphoma/leukaemia is made. His creatinine is 130 μmol/l (60–125) and his LDH is 1000 iu/l (200–450). Other screening tests show that he has sickle cell trait and G6PD deficiency. As he has stage IV Burkitt lymphoma with LDH more than twice normal he is assessed at being at high risk of tumour lysis syndrome. He is about to commence chemotherapy.

Supportive care should include:

a Intravenous fluids 3 l/m²/d
b Intravenous fluids 3 l/m²/d plus allopurinol
c Intravenous fluids 3 l/m²/d plus rasburicase
d Intravenous fluids 3 l/m²/d plus allopurinol plus urinary alkalinisation
e Intravenous fluids 3 l/m²/d plus rasburicase plus urinary alkalinisation

SBA 42

A 67-year-old woman presents with recent onset of a unilateral temporal and occipital headache. She has had one episode of double vision and on brushing her hair she has noticed that her scalp is tender. Her temperature is 38°C and she has recently lost weight. Her FBC shows an Hb of 105 g/l with an MCV of 84 fl. Her ESR is 60 mm in 1 h (<20).

You would manage the patient by:

a Administration of ibuprofen or diclofenac
b Bilateral temporal artery biopsy followed by prednisolone in a dose of 60 mg daily
c Immediate methyl prednisolone 1 g intravenously
d Immediate prednisolone in a dose of 60 mg daily
e Temporal artery biopsy followed by prednisolone in a dose of 40–60 mg daily

SBA 43

A 53-year-old Northern European Caucasian woman presents with dysphasia and weakness of the right arm lasting for 4 hours. No carotid bruit, cardiac murmur or other abnormality is detected on physical examination. A routine FBC shows WBC 13.5×10^9/l, RBC 5.96×10^{12}/l, Hb 137 g/l, Hct 0.44 l/l, MCV 74.5 fl, MCH 23 pg, MCHC 308 g/l and platelet count 512×10^9/l. Serum ferritin is 12 µg/l (12–150).

The next step in your management would be:

a Bone marrow aspiration
b High performance liquid chromatography measurement of haemoglobin A_2 percentage, suspecting β thalassaemia heterozygosity
c Measurement of serum iron and iron binding capacity
d Molecular analysis for *JAK2* mutation
e Therapeutic trial of iron

SBA 44

A 35-year-old woman with a previous history of a cerebrovascular accident presents with breathlessness, cough and a left-sided pleuritic chest pain of 1 week's duration. She is afebrile and normotensive with a mild residual hemiparesis. A chest X-ray shows a pleural-based shadow. Her FBC shows WBC $13 \times 10^9/l$, neutrophil count $11.0 \times 10^9/l$, Hb 135 g/l and platelet count $512 \times 10^9/l$. Her PT is 15 s (12–14) and APTT 50 s (26–34).

The next step in your management would be:

a Bone marrow aspirate and trephine biopsy
b Computed tomography pulmonary angiogram
c Sputum culture followed by antibiotics
d Test for lupus anticoagulant and antiphospholipid antibodies
e Ventilation–perfusion (V/Q) scan

SBA 45

A 55-year-old man presents with a history of recurrent episodes of nausea, palpitations, dizziness and flushing. He has occasionally lost consciousness. One particularly severe attack followed a bee-sting. On some occasions when he has sought urgent medical attention he has been found to be hypotensive with tachycardia and on one occasion an electrocardiogram showed mild ST depression. The patient also gives a history of indigestion. His FBC shows Hb 132 g/l, WBC $9.8 \times 10^9/l$, eosinophils $0.8 \times 10^9/l$ and monocytes $0.9 \times 10^9/l$ with neutrophil, lymphocyte and platelet counts being normal.

The next step in your management would be:

a 24-hour cardiac monitoring
b Serum IgE
c Serum tryptase
d Skin testing
e Trial of antihistamines

SBA 46

A 76-year-old woman presents with an episode of dysphasia persisting for 2 hours. She is found to have a blood pressure of 150/95 mmHg.

A $CHAD_2DS_2$-VASc score to estimate her risk of stroke is 4. A HAS-BLED score to estimate her risk of bleeding is 2.

In addition to control of her hypertension, your advice to the patient is:

a Aspirin
b No further measures needed
c Non-vitamin K antagonist oral anticoagulant (apixaban, dabigatran or rivaroxaban)
d Warfarin
e Warfarin or non-vitamin K antagonist oral anticoagulant

SBA 47

A 70-year-old woman is admitted with a left hemiparesis and aphasia. On examination, she is found to be in atrial fibrillation. A CT scan show a right cerebral haemorrhage. She is unable to give a coherent history but her husband produces a list of her medications; she is taking felodipine, irbesartan, rivaroxaban and rosuvastatin and he reports that she took all her medications as normal on the morning of admission. Laboratory tests show a platelet count of $243 \times 10^9/l$, PT 14 s (10–12) and APTT 35 s (26–40).

The correct assessment of her coagulation status is:

a Irbesartan is relevant and she is likely to be fully anticoagulated
b Irbesartan is relevant but there is no evidence of an anticoagulant effect
c None of the medications she is taking is relevant
d Rivaroxaban is relevant and she is likely to be fully anticoagulated
e Rivaroxaban is relevant but there is no evidence of an anticoagulant effect

SBA 48

A 55-year-old man with a recent diagnosis of carcinoma of the lung and pulmonary embolism has been prescribed warfarin. He presents with major gastrointestinal bleeding and an INR of 4.5.

Optimal management, in addition to red cell transfusion as indicated, is:

a Four-factor prothrombin complex
b Four-factor prothrombin complex plus vitamin K
c Fresh frozen plasma with or without vitamin K
d Recombinant activated factor VII
e Three-factor prothrombin complex plus vitamin K

SBA 49

A 55-year-old man is reviewed in pre-admission clinic prior to a hernia repair. He reports that he bled badly after tonsillectomy as a child and required blood transfusion. A coagulation screen shows PT 10.7 s (9.6–11.6) and APTT 63 s (26–32). Thrombin time is normal.

The most likely explanation is:

a Combined factor V and VIII deficiency
b Factor V deficiency
c Factor VII deficiency
d Factor XI deficiency
e Factor XII deficiency

SBA 50

A 66-year-old man has alcoholic cirrhosis but is now abstinent. He develops a strangulated inguinal hernia and requires surgery. On preoperative assessment his FBC shows WBC 7.5 × 10⁹/l, Hb 110 g/l, MCV 99 fl and platelet count 51 × 10⁹/l. His INR is 1.8.

Prior to surgery he requires:

a Fresh frozen plasma
b No specific treatment
c Platelet transfusion
d Prothrombin complex concentrate
e Vitamin K

Section 2:
Single Best Answers
Questions 51–120

This section comprises 70 Single Best Answer (SBA) multiple choice questions. They are most appropriate for haematology specialist trainees but some will be useful to core medical trainees. Normal ranges are given within parentheses. Answers and feedback will be found on pages 124–154.

Multiple Choice Questions for Haematology and Core Medical Trainees, First Edition.
Barbara J. Bain.
© 2016 John Wiley & Sons, Ltd. Published 2016 by John Wiley & Sons, Ltd.

SBA 51

A 65-year-old Afro-Caribbean woman presents with severe pruritus. She is found to have generalised erythroderma, alopecia and generalised lymphadenopathy with nodes being 1.5–3 cm in diameter. Her spleen is not palpable. FBC shows WBC 17.2 × 10⁹/l, Hb 108 g/l, neutrophils 8.8 × 10⁹/l, lymphocytes 4.5 × 10⁹/l, eosinophils 2.9 × 10⁹/l and platelets 523 × 10⁹/l. Some abnormal lymphocytes are seen and immunophenotyping shows a population of cells with the phenotype CD2–, CD3+, CD4+, CD5+, CD7– and CD25–.

The most likely diagnosis is:

a Adult T-cell leukaemia/lymphoma (ATLL)
b Idiopathic hypereosinophilic syndrome (idiopathic HES)
c Mycosis fungoides
d Sézary syndrome
e T-cell prolymphocytic leukaemia (T-PLL)

SBA 52

An 11-year-old boy presents with lethargy and weight loss. Other than pallor of the skin and conjunctivae, the only abnormality on physical examination is enlargement of the spleen 7 cm below the left costal margin. His FBC shows WBC 180 × 10⁹/l, Hb 78 g/l and platelet count 610 × 10⁹/l. His differential count shows blast cells 5%, promyelocytes 8%, myelocytes 22%, metamyelocytes 5%, neutrophils 51%, basophils 5%, eosinophils 2%, lymphocytes 1% and monocytes 1%. A bone marrow aspirate and cytogenetic and molecular genetic analysis are performed and he is commenced on allopurinol and hydroxycarbamide.

In view of your provisional diagnosis, the treatment that is likely to be indicated now is:

a Daunorubicin plus cytarabine
b Imatinib 200–300 mg daily
c Imatinib 400–600 mg daily
d Interferon alpha
e Leukapheresis

SBA 53

A 40-year-old woman presents with a 3 cm lymph node in the right supraclavicular fossa. She is asymptomatic. FBC is normal and the erythrocyte sedimentation rate (ESR) is 30 mm in 1 hour (<20). Liver function tests are normal. An excision biopsy shows nodular sclerosing Hodgkin lymphoma. Bone marrow aspirate and trephine biopsy and a combined positron emission tomography/computed tomography (PET/CT) scan show no evidence of other sites of disease.

Optimal management is:

a Combination chemotherapy
b Combination chemotherapy followed by involved field radiotherapy
c Involved field radiotherapy
d Irradiation of right and left neck and right axilla
e No further treatment indicated

SBA 54

A 67-year-old Chinese man presents with headache, dizziness and pruritus following a hot bath. On physical examination, his spleen tip is felt. His FBC shows WBC 8.7×10^9/l, Hb 200 g/l, MCV 87 fl and platelet count 250×10^9/l. Serum erythropoietin is <2.5 iu/l (4–16). Molecular analysis does not show *JAK2* V617F.

Your next step would be:

a Abdominal CT scan to look for a renal cyst or tumour
b Chest X-ray and measurement of blood gases
c Investigation for mutation in the genes encoding erythropoietin and the erythropoietin receptor
d Molecular analysis for a *CALR* (calreticulin) mutation
e Molecular analysis for a *JAK2* exon 12 mutation

SBA 55

A 3-year-old boy with no family history of a bleeding disorder presents with abdominal distension and epistaxis. Laboratory tests show Hb 82 g/l (107–137), platelet count 245 × 10^9/l (210–430), activated partial thromboplastin time (APTT) 49.2 s (26–34), prothrombin time (PT) 12.4 s (12–14), factor VIII 16% (50–150%), factor IX 74% (50–150), von Willebrand factor/ristocetin cofactor (VWF/RiCoF) 12% (50–200) and von Willebrand antigen 31% (50–200). High molecular weight VWF multimers are reduced. Magnetic resonance imaging (MRI) shows that the abdominal distension is due to a mass arising in the left kidney.

The most likely diagnosis is:

a Acquired von Willebrand disease
b Haemophilia A with haemorrhage into the kidney
c Type I von Willebrand disease
d Type IIb von Willebrand disease
e Type III von Willebrand disease

SBA 56

A 45-year-old man with paroxysmal nocturnal haemoglobinuria responds to eculizumab therapy but remains anaemic with an Hb of 92 g/l and an increased reticulocyte count and lactate dehydrogenase (LDH). His direct antiglobulin test is positive for C3 and negative for immunoglobulin (Ig) G.

The most likely explanation of the positive direct antiglobulin test is:

a He has developed a cold antibody, which is fixing complement
b He has developed warm autoimmune haemolytic anaemia
c He is becoming refractory to eculizumab
d Immune complexes resulting from development of antibodies to eculizumab are fixing complement
e The eculizumab therapy is unmasking C3 binding to red cells

SBA 57

You are discussing possible blood transfusion with a 68-year-old woman with refractory anaemia. Cytogenetic analysis has shown trisomy 8. She has not previously been transfused. She is A RhD negative and has had two pregnancies. The patient is worried about the risks of transfusion.

In current UK experience, the most likely adverse event is:

a Anaphylactic reaction
b Delayed haemolytic transfusion reaction
c Transfusion of a bacterially contaminated product
d Transfusion of blood intended for another patient
e Transmission of viral infection during the window period

SBA 58

A high platelet count (778×10^9/l) is an incidental finding in a 35-year-old woman. She is referred to haematology outpatients where she is seen 4 weeks later. There is no other relevant history and specifically nothing to suggest an infective or inflammatory disorder. Her spleen is felt on inspiration. On this occasion the platelet count is 670×10^9/l with a WBC of 11.2×10^9/l, Hb 148 g/l and MCV 97 fl. A manual differential count shows neutrophils of 9.0×10^9/l and basophils of 0.2×10^9/l. No neutrophil precursors or NRBC are seen. Erythrocyte sedimentation rate and C-reactive protein are normal. Analysis for *JAK2* V617F is therefore done and is negative.

The next thing you would do is:

a Arrange molecular analysis for a *CALR* mutation and *BCR-ABL1*
b Arrange molecular analysis for a *JAK2* exon 12 mutation
c Arrange molecular analysis for an *MPL* mutation
d Conclude that the patient has essential thrombocythaemia
e Suspect the 5q– syndrome

SBA 59

A 17-year-old man with sickle cell anaemia requires cholecystectomy. His Hb is 77 g/l. He has not been transfused or suffered from the acute chest syndrome in the last year.

Prior to surgery you would advise:

a Exchange transfusion to achieve a haemoglobin S percentage below 30%
b Exchange transfusion to achieve a haemoglobin S percentage below 50%
c No transfusion
d Top-up transfusion to achieve an Hb of 100 g/l
e Top-up transfusion to achieve an Hb of 120 g/l

SBA 60

A 67-year-old man with primary myelofibrosis associated with a *CALR* mutation has enlargement of the spleen 15 cm below the left costal margin, which is causing discomfort. He has lost weight and is suffering from fatigue. FBC shows WBC 5.4×10^9/l, Hb 85 g/l, MCV 92 fl and platelet count 70×10^9/l.

The management you would advise is:

a Hydroxycarbamide (hydroxyurea)
b Lenalidomide
c Pegylated interferon
d Ruxolitinib
e Splenectomy, preceded by appropriate vaccinations

SBA 61

A 4-year-old girl presents with marked hepatosplenomegaly, a cough, tachypnoea and a rash. Chest radiography shows interstitial infiltrates. Her FBC shows WBC $30 \times 10^9/l$, Hb 80 g/l and platelet count $70 \times 10^9/l$. A blood film is leucoerythroblastic with 1% blast cells, marked monocytosis and dysplastic features in neutrophils. Basophils are prominent. High performance liquid chromatography shows 72% haemoglobin F, 28% haemoglobin A and absent haemoglobin A_2.

The most likely diagnosis is:

a Chronic myelogenous leukaemia
b δβ thalassaemia
c Juvenile myelomonocytic leukaemia
d Leukaemoid reaction to tuberculosis
e Thalassaemia intermedia

SBA 62

A 42-year-old previously healthy woman presents with fever and pharyngitis and is found to have pancytopenia. The FBC shows WBC $3.8 \times 10^9/l$, neutrophils $0.8 \times 10^9/l$, Hb 89 g/dl and platelet count $18 \times 10^9/l$. A bone marrow aspirate is hypocellular and shows moderate dyserythropoiesis. A trephine biopsy section shows 30% cellularity with an infiltrate of lymphocytes and plasma cells, without light chain restriction. The patient has no siblings.

Optimal initial management is:

a Alemtuzumab
b Allogeneic stem cell transplantation from a volunteer unrelated donor
c Azacitidine or other hypomethylating agent
d Horse antithymocyte globulin plus ciclosporin
e Rabbit antithymocyte globulin

SBA 63

A male infant develops autoimmune thrombocytopenia at the age of 7 months. Subsequently he develops severe neutropenia and a positive direct antiglobulin test with reticulocytosis. Analysis of peripheral blood lymphocytes shows 16% of lymphocyte to be T cells expressing T-cell receptor αβ and CD3 but not CD4 or CD8. There are normal numbers of CD19+ and CD3-CD16+CD56+ lymphocytes.

The most appropriate diagnosis is:

a Autoimmune lymphoproliferative syndrome
b Common variable immunodeficiency
c Evans syndrome
d Severe combined immune deficiency (SCID)
e Systemic lupus erythematosus (SLE)

SBA 64

A 60-year-old man presents with multiple violaceous skin plaques. His FBC is normal. A biopsy is performed and shows a dermal infiltrate without epidermotropism. Immunohistochemistry shows the infiltrating cells to express CD4, CD33, CD56 and CD123.

The most likely diagnosis is:

a Blastic plasmacytoid dendritic cell neoplasm
b Granulocytic sarcoma
c Monocytic sarcoma
d NK cell lymphoma
e Peripheral T-cell lymphoma, not otherwise specified

SBA 65

A 48-year-old man whose parents were born in Jamaica presents with fever, night sweats and weight loss. On examination, he appears dehydrated but has no hepatosplenomegaly or lymphadenopathy. His FBC shows WBC $90 \times 10^9/l$, Hb 155 g/l, MCV 80 fl and platelet count $48 \times 10^9/l$. A blood film shows 80–90% abnormal lymphoid cells. On biochemical screening there is a corrected calcium of 4.35 mmol/l (2.15–2.55) and an LDH of 1,395 iu/l (200–450). Immunophenotyping shows a lymphoid population expressing CD4, CD5, CD25 and CD45. There is no expression of surface membrane CD3, CD7, CD8 or CD10.

The most likely diagnosis is:

a Adult T-cell leukaemia/lymphoma
b Angioimmunoblastic T-cell lymphoma
c Gamma-delta T-cell lymphoma
d T-lineage acute lymphoblastic leukaemia
e T-lineage prolymphocytic leukaemia

SBA 66

A 40-year-old man who has a life-long history of a bleeding disorder and a diagnosis many decades earlier of 'haemophilia' presents with a gastrointestinal haemorrhage. He has previously suffered recurrent haemarthroses, gastrointestinal and soft tissue bleeding, and bleeding following dental procedures. He has four siblings, one of whom (a brother) is similarly affected. When he initially attended outpatients 1 week earlier, the following results were obtained: PT 12 s (12–14), APTT 66 s (24–30), factor VIII 1%, von Willebrand antigen <1% and ristocetin co-factor 3%. Von Willebrand multimers were barely detectable but showed a normal range of sizes. No factor VIII inhibitor was detected.

In addition to red cell transfusion, treatment indicated is:

a Desmopressin (DDAVP)
b Pathogen-reduced fresh frozen plasma
c Recombinant human factor VIII
d Tranexamic acid
e Von Willebrand factor-containing plasma-derived concentrate

SBA 67

A 77-year-old man presents with confusion and hypercalcaemia. A CT scan shows generalised thoracic and abdominal lymphadenopathy. His FBC shows WBC 10.1 × 10⁹/l, Hb 128 g/l and platelet count 127 × 10⁹/l. A blood film shows 8% of medium-sized cells with scanty, basophilic, vacuolated cytoplasm, some with prominent nucleoli. A lymph node biopsy shows necrosis with areas of dense infiltration by medium-sized and large lymphoid cells, a high mitotic rate and apoptotic debris. The cells express CD10, CD19, CD20, BCL2 and focal, weak BCL6. Fluorescence *in situ* hybridisation (FISH) analysis shows rearrangement of *MYC* and *BCL2*. The proliferation fraction (Ki-67) is 80%.

According to the 2008 *WHO classification of Tumours of Haematopoietic and Lymphoid Tissues*, the diagnosis is:

a B-cell lymphoma, unclassifiable, with features intermediate between diffuse large B-cell lymphoma and Burkitt lymphoma
b Burkitt lymphoma
c Diffuse large B-cell lymphoma
d 'Double-hit' lymphoma
e L3 acute lymphoblastic leukaemia

SBA 68

A 72-year-old woman has a history of acrocyanosis dating back several years. She now has a symptomatic anaemia and a diagnosis of cold haemagglutinin disease has been made. She has no hepatomegaly or lymphadenopathy on physical examination or imaging but a low concentration IgM paraprotein is detected in her serum. Bone marrow aspiration and trephine biopsy find only low numbers of plasmacytoid lymphocytes.

You first choice of treatment would be:

a Chlorambucil
b Corticosteroids
c Cyclophosphamide
d Rituximab
e Splenectomy

SBA 69

A 57-year-old woman presents with redness and irritation of the right eye. On examination, there is an area of thickening and redness of the conjunctiva. A biopsy shows extranodal marginal zone (MALT-type) lymphoma.

The initial management you would advise is:

a Chlorambucil
b Culture for *Chlamydophila psittaci*
c Doxycycline
d Irradiation
e 'Watch and wait'

SBA 70

A 37-year-old man presents with fatigue and bruising. FBC shows WBC 3.8×10^9/l, neutrophils 0.9×10^9/l, Hb 77 g/l and platelet count 110×10^9/l. A bone marrow aspirate is aparticulate and hypocellular and shows minor dyserythropoiesis. A trephine biopsy shows 10% cellularity. There are hypercellular foci showing dysplastic erythropoietic cells.

A diagnosis of hypoplastic myelodysplastic syndrome (MDS) rather than aplastic anaemia would be favoured by:

a Clusters of CD34-positive cells in biopsy sections
b Cytogenetic analysis showing 47,XY,+8[2];46,XY[18]
c Low absolute reticulocyte count
d Macrocytosis
e Presence of a minor PNH clone on flow cytometry

SBA 71

A 54-year-old woman is found to have an abnormal FBC during follow-up at a breast clinic. Two years earlier she had had a mastectomy and adjuvant chemotherapy (cyclophosphamide, doxorubicin and placitaxel) for carcinoma of the breast. FBC shows WBC $2.0 \times 10^9/l$, neutrophils $0.64 \times 10^9/l$, Hb 112 g/l, MCV 105 fl and platelet count $149 \times 10^9/l$. There are dysplastic neutrophils and occasional blast cells. A bone marrow aspirate shows 12% blast cells. No Auer rods are seen. Cytogenetic analysis shows t(11;19)(q23;p13.1).

The most likely diagnosis is:

a Myelodysplastic syndrome, unclassified
b Refractory anaemia with excess of blasts 1
c Refractory anaemia with excess of blasts 2
d Refractory anaemia with multilineage dysplasia
e Therapy-related myeloid neoplasm

SBA 72

A 69-year-old man without a previous history of haemophilia is known to have a high titre factor VIII inhibitor. He presents with extensive ecchymoses and a major gastrointestinal haemorrhage.

Optimal management, in addition to red cell transfusion as indicated, is:

a Desmopressin (DDAVP) followed by cyclophosphamide
b High dose recombinant human factor VIII plus plasmapheresis with immunoadsorption
c Porcine factor VIII followed by rituximab
d Recombinant factor VIIa followed by rituximab
e Recombinant factor VIIa OR activated prothrombin complex, followed by cyclophosphamide and corticosteroids

SBA 73

A 17-year-old woman presents with microangiopathic haemolytic anaemia, hypertension, acute renal injury (creatinine 285 µmol/l) and a platelet count of 40×10^9/l. ADAMTS13 is found to be 55%. Atypical haemolytic uraemic syndrome (aHUS) is suspected.

The most effective management is likely to be:

a Haemodialysis
b Plasma exchange and immunosuppressive therapy
c Plasma exchange followed by eculizumab
d Plasma exchange until remission occurs
e Plasma exchange until remission occurs and then maintenance plasma exchange

SBA 74

A 61-year-old woman with mild type 1 von Willebrand disease required surgery for hyperparathyroidism. She was prescribed desmopressin in a dose of 17 µg (0.3 µg/kg) pre-operatively, to be repeated 24 hours post-operatively. Surgery was uneventful with no abnormal bleeding. The next morning nursing staff noted poor urine output and encouraged oral intake of fluids. The patient complained of nausea. Plasma sodium was 127 mmol/l.

Optimal management would be:

a Administration of intravenous normal saline
b Administration of recombinant factor VIII
c Continued encouragement oral fluid intake
d Withholding the second dose of desmopressin
e Withholding the second dose of desmopressin and no encouragement of oral fluid intake

SBA 75

Imatinib therapy is most likely to be of benefit in:

a Essential thrombocythaemia with a *CALR* mutation
b Chronic eosinophilic leukaemia with *PDGFRB* rearrangement
c Chronic myelomonocytic leukaemia with an *NRAS* mutation
d Chronic neutrophilic leukaemia with a *CSF3R* mutation
e Systemic mastocytosis with a *KIT* D816V mutation

SBA 76

A 59-year-old man has generalised lymphadenopathy and splenomegaly. His FBC shows WBC 98 × 10⁹/l, Hb 103 g/l, platelet count 221 × 10⁹/l, neutrophils 7.2 × 10⁹/l and lymphocytes 91 × 10⁹/l. His blood film shows mature small lymphocytes with scanty cytoplasm, round nuclei and coarsely clumped chromatin. There are some smear cells.

The tyrosine kinase inhibitor most likely to be of benefit is:

a Dasatinib
b Ibrutinib
c Imatinib
d Ponatinib
e Ruxolitinib

SBA 77

A regional flow cytometry laboratory receives a bone marrow aspirate for immunophenotyping with the clinical details given being '? acute leukaemia'. They are unable to contact the referring haematologist and so carry out immunophenotyping. This identifies a population of cells with high forward and side scatter with expression of myeloperoxidase, CD2, CD13 (heterogeneous), CD33, CD56, CD64 and CD117. There is no expression of CD34, HLA-DR or terminal deoxynucleotidyl transferase (TdT).

The most likely diagnosis is:

a Acute myeloid leukaemia with inv(16)
b Acute promyelocytic leukaemia
c Atypical chronic myeloid leukaemia
d Bilineage acute leukaemia
e Mixed phenotype acute leukaemia

SBA 78

A 39-year-old Arab woman with thalassaemia intermedia maintains an Hb around 70 g/l. She has been transfused several times during her life, during intercurrent illnesses. She had been found to have an elevated serum ferritin and has been on deferasirox for several years. Her serum ferritin is now 950 µg/l.

The next step in management is:

a Arrange magnetic resonance imaging
b Change to desferrioxamine (deferoxamine)
c Continue on same dose of deferasirox since ferritin is less than 1000 µg/l
d Increase deferasirox dose
e Perform ultrasound examination of liver

SBA 79

A 6-year-old Nigerian boy presents with Burkitt lymphoma with the presence of bulky disease and circulating lymphoma cells. He is commenced on intensive chemotherapy with allopurinol and adequate hydration. Despite this management, he develops asymptomatic biochemical abnormalities. Potassium is 5 mmol/l (3.5–5.0), uric acid 500 µmol/l (200–430), calcium 1.7 mmol/l (2.2–2.6) and creatinine 120 µmol/l (53–115). An urgent assay shows that he is glucose-6-phosphate dehydrogenase (G6PD) deficient.

In addition to maintaining hydration and careful monitoring of fluid balance and biochemical measurements, treatment indicated is:

a Continuation of allopurinol
b Haemofiltration
c Peritoneal dialysis
d Rasburicase
e Urinary alkalinisation

SBA 80

A 39-year-old woman presents with fever and mental confusion. Her FBC shows WBC 9.8 × 10⁹/l, Hb 93 g/l, platelet count 71 × 10⁹/l and reticulocytes 250 × 10⁹/l. Creatinine is 125 µmol/l. Her blood film shows polychromatic macrocytes and schistocytes. A coagulation screen is essentially normal. Urgent plasmapheresis is considered indicated

The most suitable replacement fluid is:

a 4% Gelofusine (succinylated gelatine)
b 4.5% Human Albumin Solution
c Crystalloid supplemented with cryoprecipitate if fibrinogen concentration falls
d Fresh frozen plasma
e Solvent detergent-treated fresh frozen plasma

SBA 81

A 3-year-old boy with Down syndrome presents with lymphadenopathy and is found to have B-lineage acute lymphoblastic leukaemia (ALL). Cytogenetic analysis shows 47,XY,+21c[20]. He has had correction of a congenital cardiac defect but has otherwise been well.

Optimal management is:

a Allogeneic transplantation in first remission
b High intensity treatment
c High intensity treatment followed by autologous transplantation
d Reduced intensity treatment
e Risk stratification with intensity of treatment determined by risk group

SBA 82

A 32-year-old woman who had previously suffered three miscarriages before 10 weeks of gestation is found to have a lupus anticoagulant and antibodies to β2 glycoprotein 1. The tests are repeated 12 weeks later and are still positive. One year later she falls pregnant again.

Optimal management of the pregnancy is:

a Aspirin
b Aspirin plus low molecular weight heparin
c Aspirin plus unfractionated heparin
d Corticosteroids
e Low molecular weight heparin

SBA 83

A 37-year-old man with refractory acute myeloid leukaemia receives, sequentially, chemotherapy and a sibling haemopoietic stem cell transplantation. He becomes febrile and requires antibiotics. Two weeks after the transplant he is again febrile and in addition is jaundiced and hypotensive. FBC shows WBC 0.2×10^9/l, Hb 71 g/l and platelet count 82×10^9/l. His blood film shows spherocytes, microspherocytes and polychromatic macrocytes.

The most likely diagnosis is:

a Alloimmune haemolytic anaemia
b Autoimmune haemolytic anaemia
c *Clostridium perfringens* sepsis
d Hereditary spherocytosis
e Microangiopathic haemolytic anaemia

SBA 84

A patient who has been receiving dabigatran requires emergency surgery under spinal anaesthesia.

The presence of a clinically significant level of the drug can be excluded by:

a A normal activated partial thromboplastin time (APTT)
b A normal activated whole blood clotting time
c A normal prothrombin time (PT)
d A normal thrombin time
e Protamine neutralisation assay

SBA 85

A 39-year-old pregnant woman presents with bilateral breast masses and cervical lymphadenopathy. FBC is normal. A biopsy shows a tumour with many mitotic figures and apoptotic cells. The tumour cells express CD10, CD20 and BCL6 but not TdT. Ki-67 is expressed in 99% of cells.

The most likely genetic abnormality is:

a Presence of *BCR-ABL1*
b Mutation in *BRAC1*
c Rearrangement of *BCL2*
d Rearrangement of *BCL6*
e Rearrangement of *MYC*

SBA 86

A 9-year-old boy presents with the recent onset of bruising and is found to also have petechiae and bleeding from his mouth. There is no other abnormality on physical examination. His FBC shows an Hb of 109 g/l and a platelet count of 8×10^9/l. His blood film confirms the count and is otherwise normal. His blood group is O RhD positive.

Optimal initial management is:

a Anti-D
b Bone marrow aspiration to exclude acute lymphoblastic leukaemia
c Careful observation
d High dose intravenous immunoglobulin
e Oral corticosteroids

SBA 87

A 3-year-old boy presents with a rash and polyuria and is found to have diabetes insipidus. He has enlarged cervical lymph nodes and several palpable masses overlying defects in his skull. Haemoglobin concentration is 67 g/l with features of anaemia of chronic disease. A biopsy of a soft tissue mass is performed.

The immunophenotypic marker that would confirm the diagnosis you are suspecting is:

a ALK1
b CD1a
c CD3
d CD38
e CD138

SBA 88

A 10-year-old girl with chronic anaemia has had a poor response to oral iron therapy. Her FBC shows RBC 3.37×10^{12}/l, Hb 58 g/l, Hct 0.21 l/l, MCV 61.8 fl, MCH 17.2 pg and MCHC 279 g/l. Other tests show serum iron 2.04 µmol/l (11–28), transferrin saturation 7% (12–45), serum ferritin 143 µg/l (14–200) and serum hepcidin 11.96 nmol/l (1.4–5.5).

The most likely diagnosis is:

a Anaemia of chronic disease
b Congenital sideroblastic anaemia
c Iron deficiency due to chronic occult blood loss
d Iron deficiency due to coeliac disease
e Iron-refractory iron deficiency anaemia

SBA 89

A 16-year-old boy appears to be lacking in energy. There is no abnormality on physical examination and no relevant family history. His FBC shows Hb 103 g/l and MCV 67 fl. His blood film is dimorphic. A bone marrow aspirate shows numerous ring sideroblasts and he is found to have a mutation in *ALAS2*. Serum ferritin is 1100 µg/l (14–200).

Your **initial** management would be:

a Ascorbic acid
b Erythropoietin
c Phlebotomy to normalise iron stores
d Pyridoxine 10 mg daily
e Pyridoxine 200 mg daily

SBA 90

A 48-year-old woman with poor prognosis myelodysplastic syndrome receives an allogeneic haemopoietic stem cell transplant from a matched unrelated donor after conditioning with busulphan and cyclophosphamide. She then receives sirolimus and methotrexate as prophylaxis against graft-versus-host disease. A week after transplantation she develops abdominal pain and respiratory distress and is found to have gained weight. On examination, her liver is tender and she has oedema and ascites. Her bilirubin has risen to 154 µmol/l and alanine aminotransferase is greatly elevated. Creatinine has risen to 200 µmol/l.

Given the most likely diagnosis, the treatment you would advise is:

a Cautious paracentesis and defibrotide
b Heparin
c Paracentesis and vigorous diuretic therapy
d Tissue plasminogen activator
e Vigorous diuretic therapy

SBA 91

The pathogenesis of anaemia of chronic disease is complex but involves hepcidin.

In this condition, hepcidin is:

a Decreased as a result of increased secretion of interleukin 6 by inflammatory cells
b Decreased leading to impaired mobilisation of hepatic iron
c Decreased leading to impaired release of iron from macrophages
d Increased leading to a fall in transferrin concentration
e Increased leading to impaired release of iron from macrophages and reduced delivery of iron into the plasma by enterocytes

SBA 92

A 39-year-old man who has previously has a renal transplant presents with cognitive impairment and a seizure. MRI with gadolinium contrast shows an enhancing tumour mass in the left cerebral hemisphere with surrounding oedema. A stereotactic brain biopsy shows a diffuse large B-cell lymphoma with an activated B-cell phenotype. There is no evidence of disease outside the central nervous system.

Optimal management is:

a Dexamethasone followed by high dose methotrexate
b High dose methotrexate followed by dose-intensive consolidation chemotherapy
c Surgery followed by whole brain irradiation
d Whole brain irradiation
e Whole brain irradiation plus intrathecal methotrexate

SBA 93

A 70-year-old woman is taking dabigatran for atrial fibrillation detected after she suffered a cerebrovascular accident. She re-presents with a gastrointestinal haemorrhage and an assessment of plasma concentration of dabigatran is required.

The recommended test is:

a Activated partial thromboplastin time (APTT)
b Chromogenic assay for anti-thrombin activity
c Prothrombin time (PT)
d Reptilase time
e Thromboelastogram

SBA 94

A 60-year-old 100-kg woman who has had bariatric surgery presents with numbness in her hands and feet and unsteady gait. She has a past history of carpal tunnel syndrome and treated hypothyroidism. Her FBC shows Hb 103 g/l, MCV 103 fl, neutrophil count 0.5×10^9/l and platelet count 120×10^9/l. A bone marrow aspirate shows vacuolation of haemopoietic precursors and small numbers of ring sideroblasts.

The most likely diagnosis is:

a Copper deficiency
b Hypothyroidism
c Myelodysplastic syndrome
d Pyridoxine deficiency
e Vitamin B_{12} deficiency

SBA 95

A 23-year-old Sicilian woman present to the antenatal clinic at 14 weeks of gestation. Her FBC shows RBC 4.77 × 10^{12}/l, Hb 103 g/l, MCV 70 fl, Hct 0.33 l/l, MCH 21.9 pg, MCHC 311 g/l and reticulocyte count 6%. Haemoglobinopathy investigations show haemoglobin A 10%, haemoglobin S 79%, haemoglobin F 5% and haemoglobin A_2 4.9%. Her partner is also Sicilian.

With regard to the pregnancy outcome, the most relevant finding in her partner would be:

a α^0 thalassaemia heterozygosity
b β thalassaemia heterozygosity
c Haemoglobin H disease
d Heterozygosity for either β thalassaemia or haemoglobin S
e Sickle cell heterozygosity

SBA 96

A 5-year-old girl presents with pallor and splenomegaly (spleen felt 3 cm below left costal margin). Her FBC shows WBC 24 × 10^9/l, Hb 96 g/l, MCV 90 fl, neutrophils 7.0 × 10^9/l, lymphocytes 3.2 × 10^9/l, monocytes 12.0 × 10^9/l, eosinophils 1.3 × 10^9/l, basophils 0.5 × 10^9/l and platelets 30 × 10^9/l. A blood film confirms the platelet count and shows immature monocytes and mild granulocyte dysplasia. Haemoglobin F is found to be 45% and haemoglobin A_2 is 1%.

Optimal management is:

a Daunorubicin plus cytarabine
b Haemopoietic stem cell transplantation
c Haemopoietic stem cell transplantation preceded by chemotherapy
d Mercaptopurine
e 'Watch and wait' as spontaneous resolution may occur

SBA 97

A 65-year-old woman has a history of polycythaemia vera treated for the last 7 years with hydroxycarbamide and aspirin. She has now developed symptomatic anaemia that has not responded to cessation of hydroxycarbamide. Her spleen is palpable 2 cm below the left costal margin. A blood film is leucoerythroblastic with teardrop poikilocytes but without any dysplastic features. A bone marrow aspirate fails and a trephine biopsy shows collagen deposition. FBC shows WBC $5.2 \times 10^9/l$, Hb 72 g/l, MCV 92 fl and platelet count $78 \times 10^9/l$. Serum erythropoietin is 150 mu/ml (2.6–18.5).

The treatment most likely to be of benefit would be:

a Blood transfusion
b Danazol
c Darbepoetin
d Ruxolitinib
e Splenectomy

SBA 98

A 24-year-old Thai woman attends her general practitioner because she is planning a pregnancy and has heard that some of her cousins in Thailand have had thalassaemia. Her FBC shows an Hb of 110 g/l and an MCV of 65 fl. Her blood film is reported as showing hypochromia, microcytosis and occasional target cells and irregularly contracted cells. High performance liquid chromatography shows haemoglobin E plus A_2 to be 18.5%. Haemoglobin electrophoresis on cellulose acetate at alkaline pH confirms the presence of haemoglobin E.

The recommended next action is:

a Advise the patient that she has haemoglobin E heterozygosity and no further testing is indicated
b DNA analysis for α^0 thalassaemia
c Measure haemoglobin A_2 percentage by capillary electrophoresis
d Serum ferritin assay
e Test for haemoglobin H inclusions

SBA 99

A 23-year-old Thai woman presents to the antenatal clinic at 16 weeks gestation. FBC shows Hb 110 g/l, MCV 78 fl and MCH 26.5 pg. High performance liquid chromatography shows her to have 30% haemoglobin A_2 plus E. Screening of her partner is requested.

The most significant abnormality in her partner would be:

a α^+ thalassaemia heterozygosity
b α^0 thalassaemia heterozygosity
c β thalassaemia heterozygosity
d Haemoglobin E heterozygosity.
e Haemoglobin E homozygosity

SBA 100

A 70-year-old woman with a history of treated hypothyroidism presents with fatigue. Her FBC shows Hb 81 g/l, MCV 110 fl, neutrophil count 3.2×10^9/l and platelet count 110×10^9/l. Red cell distribution width (RDW) is increased. Bilirubin and LDH are increased.

The most specific test supporting the diagnosis you suspect would be:

a Intrinsic factor antibodies
b Parietal cell antibodies
c Red cell folate assay
d Serum holotranscobalamin assay
e Serum vitamin B_{12} assay

SBA 101

A 2-day-old baby requires an exchange transfusion for RhD haemolytic disease of the newborn. He did not require intrauterine transfusion.

In addition to being of an appropriate ABO and RhD group, the blood provided should be:

a Less than 5 days old, CMV-negative
b Less than 5 days old, CMV-negative, taken into SAG-M (saline, adenine, glucose, mannitol)
c Less than 5 days old, CMV-negative, taken into citrate-phosphate-dextrose (CPD), irradiated
d Less than 10 days old, irradiated, CMV negative
e Less than 10 days old, taken into SAG-M, irradiated

SBA 102

A 50-year-old woman presents with peripheral neuropathy, predominantly motor. She has a mass over her left buttock and splenomegaly. Her FBC shows WBC 7.2×10^9/l, Hb 129 g/l and platelet count 720×10^9/l. The mass is biopsied and demonstrated to be an IgA lambda-expressing plasmacytoma. Further investigations are therefore performed. Serum immunoglobulins are present in normal concentrations but there is a low level IgA lambda paraprotein. A lumbar puncture shows increased protein concentration but no abnormal cells. Bone marrow aspiration shows 2% plasma cells and increased megakaryocytes. A skeletal survey shows several sclerotic lesions but no osteolytic lesions.

The most appropriate diagnosis is:

a Light chain-associated amyloidosis
b Monoclonal gammopathy of undetermined significance (MGUS)
c Multiple myeloma (plasma cell myeloma)
d POEMS syndrome
e Solitary plasmacytoma

SBA 103

A 65-year-old man is found to have an abnormal blood count during follow up for his hypertension. He has a past history of myocardial infarction seven years previously. He does not smoke and is teetotal. On examination, his spleen is felt 12 cm below the left costal margin. His FBC shows WBC $12.2 \times 10^9/l$, Hb 187 g/l, Hct 0.58 and platelet count $513 \times 10^9/l$. Serum erythropoietin is reduced and bone marrow examination shows trilineage hyperplasia.

The treatment you advise is:

a Aspirin plus venesection aiming for a Hct of <0.50
b Aspirin, venesection and hydroxycarbamide
c Hydroxycarbamide
d Venesection aiming for a Hct of <0.45
e Venesection aiming for a Hct of <0.50

SBA 104

A neonate with Down syndrome is found to have hepatosplenomegaly and a violaceous skin infiltrate. Her FBC shows WBC $27.2 \times 10^9/l$, Hb 139 g/l and platelet count $27 \times 10^9/l$. A blood film shows blast cells, some of which have basophilic cytoplasm and cytoplasmic blebs, and are thought likely to be megakaryoblasts. There are occasional micromegakaryocytes, nucleated red cells and granulocyte precursors. It is concluded that the skin lesion is *leukaemia cutis*.

The most appropriate management is:

a Corticosteroids
b Cytarabine and daunorubicin
c Observation
d Platelet transfusion
e Red cell and platelet transfusion

SBA 105

A 3-month-old baby has a 'group and save' and antibody screen performed prior to cardiac surgery for cyanotic congenital heart disease. His FBC shows WBC $14.5 \times 10^9/l$, Hb 150 g/l, neutrophil count $5.6 \times 10^9/l$ and lymphocyte count $8.4 \times 10^9/l$. His red blood cells type as O RhD negative but no anti-A or anti-B is detected. A direct antiglobulin test is negative.

The interpretation of the serology is:

a Immune deficiency associated with Down syndrome
b Normal for age
c Probable human immunodeficiency virus (HIV) infection
d Probable hypogammaglobulinaemia
e Probable severe combined immune deficiency

SBA 106

A 47-year-old Northern European Caucasian woman with dermatitis herpetiformis is being treated with dapsone. She presents to Accident and Emergency having noted that her lips and fingers are blue. She has tachycardia but blood pressure is normal. Oxygen saturation measured by pulse oximetry is found to be 85% and this is confirmed on arterial blood gas analysis. Further investigation shows oxyhaemoglobin of 77% and 20% methaemoglobin.

The most appropriate management is:

a Admission to intensive care ward and administration of oxygen
b Exchange transfusion
c Intravenous methylene blue
d Observation of vital signs but no active management
e Testing for glucose-6-phosphate dehydrogenase (G6PD) deficiency before deciding on further management

SBA 107

A 65-year-old man who is receiving unfractionated heparin following major orthopaedic surgery suffers a deep vein thrombosis and a pulmonary embolus six days post-operatively. A diagnosis of heparin-induced thrombocytopenia (HIT) is established. He has been on warfarin for one day. His platelet count is 72×10^9/l.

The most appropriate management, in addition to stopping unfractionated heparin, is:

a Administration of low molecular weight heparin
b Commencement of argatroban
c Commencement of argatroban and administration of vitamin K
d Commencement of fondaparinux
e Continuation of warfarin

SBA 108

An 8-month-old Chinese baby presents with anaemia and gross hepatosplenomegaly. Her FBC shows WBC 10×10^9/l, Hb 74 g/l and platelet count 65×10^9/l. Her blood film shows anisocytosis, poikilocytosis and microcytosis. Haemoglobin electrophoresis shows 98% haemoglobin F and 1.8% haemoglobin A_2. Her father has microcytosis and a haemoglobin A_2 of 5.2%. Her mother has a normal Hb, microcytosis, haemoglobin F of 14.1% and haemoglobin A_2 of 2.4%. The baby becomes transfusion dependent.

The most likely diagnosis is:

a Compound heterozygosity for β^0 thalassaemia and $\delta\beta$ thalassaemia
b Compound heterozygosity for β^+ thalassaemia and $\delta\beta$ thalassaemia
c Compound heterozygosity for β^0 thalassaemia and hereditary persistence of fetal haemoglobin
d Homozygosity for β^0 thalassaemia
e Homozygosity for hereditary persistence of fetal haemoglobin

SBA 109

A 77-year-old man presents with a past history of deep vein thrombosis and one episode of pulmonary embolism 5 years previously. He is on long-term maintenance treatment with warfarin with his international normalised ratio (INR) being kept between 2 and 3.5. He requires cataract surgery.

The most appropriate management is:

a Change to a prophylactic dose of low molecular weight heparin
b Change to a therapeutic dose of low molecular weight heparin
c Continue warfarin at the same dose as long as the INR is in the therapeutic range
d Reduce warfarin to achieve an INR between 1.5 and 2.0
e Stop warfarin and resume several days postoperatively

SBA 110

A 69-year-old man with chronic lymphocytic leukaemia (CLL) has relapsed following treatment with fludarabine, cyclophosphamide and rituximab (FCR). His FBC shows WBC 119.2×10^9/l, lymphocytes 112.6×10^9/l, Hb 115 g/l and platelet count 120×10^9/l

Contra-indicated vaccines include:

a *Haemophilus influenza*
b Herpes zoster
c Meningococcus
d Pneumococcus
e Seasonal influenza

SBA 111

A 25-year-old woman is found in the antenatal clinic to be heterozygous for haemoglobin S.

The abnormality of most concern if found in her husband would be:

a α^0 thalassaemia
b Deletional hereditary persistence of fetal haemoglobin
c Haemoglobin E trait
d Haemoglobin D-Punjab trait
e Haemoglobin G-Philadelphia

SBA 112

A 50-year-old woman with a confirmed diagnosis of polycythaemia vera has been treated with venesection followed by hydroxycarbamide. Her FBC shows WBC 7.2×10^9/l, Hb 154 g/l, Hct 0.48 and platelet count 500×10^9/l. She complains of thinning of her hair and a rash since commencing hydroxycarbamide and is unwilling to take a higher dose.

The most appropriate management in addition to the aspirin that she is already taking would be:

a A lower dose of hydroxycarbamide
b A lower dose of hydroxycarbamide plus venesection
c Busulphan, pipobroman or ^{32}P
d Interferon
e Ruxolitinib

SBA 113

A 50-year-old woman with chronic warm autoimmune haemolytic anaemia (AIHA) has haemolysis that is refractory to prednisolone in a dose of 40 mg daily. Her Hb is 67 g/l. She has developed osteoporosis with some loss of height despite administration of calcium, vitamin D and a bisphosphonate and has impaired glucose tolerance. She is taking folic acid 5 mg daily.

Optimal management now is:

a Alemtuzumab 10 mg daily for 7–10 days
b Appropriate vaccinations followed by splenectomy
c Prednisolone in an increased dose of 60 mg daily
d Mycophenolate mofetil starting with a dose of 500 mg bd
e Rituximab in a dose of 375 mg/m^2 weekly for 4 weeks

SBA 114

A 55-year-old woman presents with bone pain and fatigue. A bone marrow aspirate shows 37% plasma cells. FISH analysis is carried out.

A better prognosis is indicated by:

a amp1q21
b del(17p13)/loss of TP53
c Hyperdiploidy
d t(4;14)(p16.3;q32)
e t(14;16)(q32;q23)

SBA 115

A 21-year-old man presents with episodic pallor, jaundice and dark urine following exercise. His FBC shows Hb 151 g/l, MCV 103 fl and MCHC 356 g/l (325-352). Reticulocytes are 5% and total and non-conjugated bilirubin are increased. Osmotic fragility is reduced and red cells show an increased sodium and reduced potassium concentration. A blood film shows occasional target cells and irregularly contracted cells.

The most likely diagnosis is:

a Familial pseudohyperkalaemia
b Hereditary pyropoikilocytosis
c Hereditary spherocytosis
d Hereditary stomatocytosis
e Hereditary xerocytosis

SBA 116

A 50-year-old woman under regular follow-up following a previous carcinoma of the breast is found on a routine blood count to have marked thrombocytosis. There are no abnormal physical findings other than the evidence of previous partial mastectomy. Her FBC shows WBC 11.2×10^9/l, Hb 151 g/l, MCV 86 fl and platelet count 1900×10^9/l. A bone marrow aspirate is normocellular with markedly increased megakaryocytes, which are reduced in size with hypolobated nuclei.

The most likely genetic abnormality is:

a BCR-ABL1
b CALR mutation
c JAK2 exon 12 mutation
d JAK2 V617F
e MPL mutation

SBA 117

A 45-year-old man who presents with stage IVB diffuse large B-cell lymphoma is found to be HIV positive. His CD4 lymphocyte count is 200/mm³ (500–1,200). Serology for hepatitis B is negative.

Optimal management is:

a Combination chemotherapy plus intrathecal methotrexate
b Highly active antiretroviral treatment (HAART), avoiding chemotherapy until immune reconstitution has occurred
c Intensive combination chemotherapy, avoiding rituximab
d Intensive combination chemotherapy plus rituximab
e Intensive combination chemotherapy plus rituximab plus HAART

SBA 118

You receive a phone call from the antenatal clinic about a patient of Greek ethnic origin who is 16 weeks pregnant. The laboratory has reported that the patient is heterozygous for haemoglobin O-Arab and the midwife wants your advice as to what to do. The patient's Hb is 122 g/l and MCV 82 fl.

The advice you give is:

a In view of the woman's ethnic origin, the variant haemoglobin has probably been misidentified
b The only significance is possible interaction with haemoglobin S
c The patient is already at 16 weeks of gestation so there is no point in any further investigation
d This variant haemoglobin can interact adversely with haemoglobin S and β thalassaemia
e This variant haemoglobin is of no significance so no further action is needed

SBA 119

A 70-year-old man presents with backache and lethargy. His FBC shows Hb 89 g/l, MCV 102 fl, WBC 46.7 × 10⁹/l, neutrophils 40.5 × 10⁹/l, myelocytes 3.6 × 10⁹/l, monocytes 0.8 × 10⁹/l and lymphocytes 1.8 × 10⁹/l. His blood film shows toxic granulation, Döhle bodies and marked rouleaux formation. He is investigated further and is found to have an IgG paraprotein in a concentration of 40 g/l

The most likely explanation of the leucocyte abnormalities is:

a Atypical chronic myeloid leukaemia
b Chronic myelogenous leukaemia
c Chronic neutrophilic leukaemia
d Neutrophilic variant of chronic myelogenous leukaemia
e Neutrophilic leukaemoid reaction

SBA 120

A 35-year-old woman presents with fatigue and abdominal discomfort. There is no relevant past medical history. She smokes 25 cigarettes a day, takes 2–3 units of alcohol on most days and has several tattoos. On examination there is no lymphadenopathy but her spleen is felt 2 cm below the left costal margin. Her FBC shows WBC 15.7 × 10⁹/l, lymphocytes 9.8 × 10⁹/l, Hb 127 g/l and platelet count 327 × 10⁹/l. Her blood film shows a significant proportion of binucleated lymphocytes and also lymphocytes with two lobes joined by a fine filament. Other lymphocytes are larger than normal and have moderately basophilic cytoplasm.

The most likely diagnosis is:

a Chronic active Epstein–Barr virus infection
b Chronic lymphocytic leukaemia
c Hepatitis C infection
d Persistent polyclonal B lymphocytosis
e Splenic marginal zone lymphoma

Section 3:
Extended Matching Questions 1–30

This section comprises 30 extended matching questions (EMQs) suitable for trainees sitting the part 1 FRCPath examination. In this section, each option from the alphabetical list can be used once, more than once or not at all. Answers will be found on pages 155–182.

Multiple Choice Questions for Haematology and Core Medical Trainees, First Edition.
Barbara J. Bain.
© 2016 John Wiley & Sons, Ltd. Published 2016 by John Wiley & Sons, Ltd.

EMQ 1

For each clinicopathological description, select the most likely diagnosis from the alphabetical list.

a Adult T-cell leukaemia/lymphoma
b Aggressive NK-cell leukaemia
c Anaplastic large cell lymphoma
d Angioimmunoblastic T-cell lymphoma
e EBV-positive T-cell lymphoproliferative disorder
f Extranodal NK/T-cell lymphoma
g Peripheral T-cell lymphoma, not otherwise specified
h T-cell large granular lymphocytic leukaemia
i T-cell precursor lymphoblastic leukaemia/lymphoma
j T-cell prolymphocytic leukaemia

(i) An 83-year old Afro-American presents with a 2-month history of weakness and malaise; he has generalised lymphadenopathy with nodes up to 2 cm in diameter. FBC shows WBC 112 × 10^9/l, lymphocyte count 99.8 × 10^9/l, Hb 108 g/l and platelet count 170 × 10^9/l; the lymphocytes are medium sized with moderately basophilic cytoplasm and a single medium sized nucleolus. Trephine biopsy sections show a heavy interstitial infiltrate with several non-paratrabecular focal accumulations. Immunophenotyping shows expression of CD2, CD3, CD4, CD5 and CD7; CD8 and terminal deoxynucleotidyl transferase (TdT) are not expressed. There is a complex karyotype including inv(14)(q11q32).

(ii) A 59-year-old Caucasian man presents with skin nodules and lymphadenopathy. A lymph node biopsy shows replacement by lymphoid cells with moderately abundant pale cytoplasm. They express CD3, CD4, CD5, CD10 and CD279. There are also some CD20-positive lymphocytes and immunoblasts. There is a mild increase in Epstein–Barr virus (EBV)-positive lymphocytes.

(iii) A 68-year-old Chinese woman complains of nasal obstruction and is found to have a lesion of the nose, which on computed tomography (CT) scanning is demonstrated to be extending into the sinuses. A biopsy shows a diffuse angiocentric, angiodestructive lymphomatous infiltrate with mucosal ulceration. The lymphoma cells express CD2, CD56, CD3ε and EBV-encoded RNA (EBER).

(iv) A 38-year-old Haitian man presents with an altered mental state. He has moderate cervical and inguinal lymphadenopathy. Laboratory tests show Hb 167 g/l, neutrophil count 15.7 × 10⁹/l, lymphocyte count 5.2 × 10⁹/l and platelet count 25 × 10⁹/l; there is hypercalcaemia, a very high lactate dehydrogenase and abnormal liver function tests. Prothrombin time is prolonged and flow cytometry shows a population of lymphocytes expressing CD3, CD4 and CD25 with partial expression of CD5 and CD8 and no expression of CD7.

(v) A 10-year-old boy presents with cervical lymphadenopathy. His blood count is normal. Lymph node biopsy shows a diffuse infiltrate of medium sized lymphoid cells with admixed macrophages giving a 'starry sky' appearance. Immunohistochemistry shows expression of CD3, CD4, CD5, CD7, CD8 and TdT.

EMQ 2

For each clinical description select the most appropriate initial treatment from the alphabetical list.

a Desmopressin
b Factor XI concentrate
c Fibrinogen concentrate
d Fibrinogen concentrate or solvent-detergent treated fresh frozen plasma
e Pathogen-reduced cryoprecipitate
f Prothrombin complex concentrate
g Recombinant activated factor VII
h Recombinant factor V
i Solvent-detergent treated fresh frozen plasma
j Tranexamic acid

(i) A neonate suffers from bleeding from the umbilical cord and subsequently becomes drowsy and is found to have suffered an intracerebral haemorrhage. Fibrinogen concentration is 0.1 g/l.

(ii) A 56-year-old man suffers a major gastrointestinal haemorrhage and is found to have a factor VII concentration of 0.01 iu/ml.

(iii) A 33-year-old woman suffers from persistent bleeding from a cut to her leg after a fall. She is known to have factor XI deficiency with levels of 0.2–0.3 iu/ml.

(iv) A 70-year-old man with factor V deficiency with a factor level of 0.1 iu/ml requires hip replacement.

(v) A 66-year-old man suffers a significant gastrointestinal haemorrhage and requires transfusion. He is known to have factor XI deficiency with levels of around 0.25 iu/ml.

EMQ 3

For each transfusion reaction select the most likely explanation from the alphabetical list.

a Acute haemolytic transfusion reaction
b Anaphylactic transfusion reaction
c Delayed haemolytic transfusion reaction
d Passenger lymphocyte syndrome
e Post-transfusion purpura
f Septic transfusion reaction
g Transfusion-associated acute lung injury (TRALI)
h Transfusion-associated circulatory overload (TACO)
i Transfusion-associated graft-versus-host disease
j Transmission of prion disease

(i) An adverse effect of transfusion the prevalence of which is related to administration of a blood component with a high content of plasma; most often due to anti-HLA antibodies.

(ii) Most often due to ABO incompatibility and may present with fever, chills, chest pain or hypotension.

(iii) Can result from anti-immunoglobulin (Ig) A or anti-haptoglobin antibodies.

(iv) Platelet concentrates are most often responsible.

(v) Usually results from re-exposure to an antigen to which the patient has already been immunised but where no antibody was detectable.

EMQ 4

For each clinical description select the most likely disease mechanism/ pathogenesis from the alphabetical list.

a Catastrophic antiphospholipid syndrome
b Cobalamin C deficiency
c Disseminated intravascular coagulation
d Drug-induced microangiopathy, dose related
e Drug-induced microangiopathy, immune
f Haemolytic uraemic syndrome
g HELLP (haemolysis, elevated liver enzymes, low platelets) syndrome
h Hereditary thrombotic thrombocytopenic purpura
i Severe sepsis
j Thrombotic thrombocytopenic purpura

   (i) A 65-year-old woman who has a history of hypertension and hypercholesterolaemia is taking enalapril and atorvastatin. She develops leg cramps and quinine is prescribed. Shortly afterwards she develops acute kidney injury and a microangiopathic haemolytic anaemia with thrombocytopenia. She is severely oliguric. ADAMTS13 is 15%.

   (ii) A 38-year-old woman presents with confusion and is found to have microangiopathic haemolytic anaemia, thrombocytopenia and a creatinine of 150 μmol/l. ADAMTS13 is 8%.

   (iii) A 35-year-old man who is receiving tacrolimus following a renal transplant develops a microangiopathic haemolytic anaemia. Platelet count is $89 \times 10^9/l$.

   (iv) A 6-year-old boy develops acute kidney injury following a school trip. FBC shows Hb 80 g/l, MCV 105 fl, platelet count $100 \times 10^9/l$ and reticulocyte count $200 \times 10^9/l$.

   (v) A newborn baby is noted to be jaundiced and investigation shows a microangiopathic haemolytic anaemia and thrombocytopenia. White cell count and MCV are normal. He is afebrile and otherwise appears well.

EMQ 5

For each clinical description select the most likely diagnosis from the list of options.

a Alloimmune thrombocytopenia
b Autoimmune thrombocytopenia (ITP)
c Bernard–Soulier syndrome
d *GATA1* mutation
e Glanzmann thrombasthenia
f *MYH9*-related disease
g Pseudo-von Willebrand disease
h Sitosterolaemia
i Von Willebrand disease
j Wiskott–Aldrich syndrome

(i) A 45-year-old man is referred for investigation of a platelet count of $45 \times 10^9/l$. He has severe bilateral sensorineural deafness. He has no bleeding tendency. A blood film shows large platelets with no definite neutrophil inclusions. His son is also found to have macrothrombocytopenia.

(ii) A 12-year-old girl whom has previously been diagnosed with idiopathic autoimmune thrombocytopenia suffers severe menorrhagia at the menarche. Her FBC shows WBC $7.2 \times 10^9/l$, Hb 72 g/l, MCV 96 fl and platelet count $36 \times 10^9/l$. Her blood film shows giant platelets and polychromasia.

(iii) An otherwise healthy neonate is noted to have petechiae and is found to have a platelet count of $15 \times 10^9/l$. His blood group is O RhD negative. His mother has a normal blood count and her blood group is A RhD negative.

(iv) A 35-year-old pregnant woman is investigated because of microcytosis and is found to be heterozygous for β thalassaemia. In addition she is found to have a platelet count of $54 \times 10^9/l$. Her neutrophils show large blue-grey inclusions.

(v) An 8-month-old boy presents with eczema and is found to have thrombocytopenia and lymphopenia. His blood film shows small platelets. No leucocyte inclusions are detected.

EMQ 6

For each clinical description select the most appropriate initial treatment plan in a patient with classical Hodgkin lymphoma.

a Antiretroviral therapy plus six cycles of ABVD (doxorubicin, bleomycin, vincristine, dacarbazine)
b Antiretroviral therapy plus six cycles of either ABVD or escalated BEACOPP (bleomycin, etoposide, doxorubicin, cyclophosphamide, vincristine, procarbazine, prednisone)
c Four courses of ABVD followed by 30 Gy radiotherapy
d Involved field radiotherapy
e Involved site radiotherapy
f Mantle radiotherapy
g Six courses of ABVD
h Six courses of ABVD or escalated BEACOPP
i Total nodal irradiation
j Two courses of ABVD followed by 20 Gy radiotherapy

   (i)   A 38-year-old man with stage IIA (left cervical and left axillary) favourable prognosis Hodgkin lymphoma.

   (ii)   A 35-year old woman with bulky mediastinal lymphadenopathy, bilateral cervical lymphadenopathy, night sweats and an erythrocyte sedimentation rate (ESR) of 55 mm in 1 h.

   (iii) A 42-year-old woman with Hodgkin lymphoma involving bilateral cervical, axillary and inguinal nodes with fevers reaching 38–39°C.

   (iv)   A 67-year-old man with stage IIIB Hodgkin lymphoma who is otherwise fit.

   (v)   A 38-year-old man who presents with stage IV Hodgkin lymphoma and is found to be HIV positive.

EMQ 7

For each lymphoma listed, select the most likely aetiological agent. Each option can be used once, more than once or not at all.

a *Achromobacter xylosoxidans*
b *Borrelia burgdorferi*
c *Campylobacter jejuni*
d *Chlamydophila psittaci*
e Epstein–Barr virus
f Epstein–Barr virus plus malaria
g *Helicobacter heilmannii*
h *Helicobacter pylori*
i Hepatitis C
j JC virus

(i) HIV-associated intracerebral diffuse large B-cell lymphoma.

(ii) *H. pylori*-negative gastric mucosa-associated lymphoid tissue (MALT)-type lymphoma.

(iii) Splenic marginal zone lymphoma (splenic lymphoma with villous lymphocytes).

(iv) Lacrimal gland MALT lymphoma.

(v) Cutaneous MALT-type lymphoma.

EMQ 8

For each clinical description select the most likely diagnosis from the alphabetical list. Each option can be used once, more than once or not at all. Age- and gender-appropriate normal ranges are given in parentheses.

a α^+ thalassaemia heterozygosity
b α^+ thalassaemia homozygosity
c β thalassaemia heterozygosity
d Acquired sideroblastic anaemia
e Anaemia of chronic disease
f Congenital sideroblastic anaemia
g Functional iron deficiency
h Iron deficiency anaemia
i Iron deficiency plus anaemia of chronic disease
j Lead poisoning

(i) A 3-year-old Caucasian boy appears tired and an FBC shows Hb 85 g/l (107–133), MCV 65 fl (73–90), MCH 20 pg (24–34), serum iron 6 μmol/l (14–33) and total iron binding capacity 80 μmol/l (45–75).

(ii) A 23-year-old Italian woman has routine testing during the first trimester of pregnancy. Her FBC shows RBC $4.39 \times 10^{12}/l$ (3.52–4.52), Hb 110 g/l (110–143), Hct 0.32 l/l (0.31–0.41), MCV 74 fl (81–96), MCH 25.2 pg (27–33), MCHC 332 (316–349) g/l. Haemoglobin A_2 is 4.4% (2.5–3.5).

(iii) A 65-year-old Afro-Caribbean woman with ulcerative colitis has an FBC that shows RBC $4.22 \times 10^{12}/l$ (3.88–4.99), Hb 70 g/l (118–148), Hct 0.29 l/l (0.36–0.44). MCV 67 fl (82–98), MCH 16.6 pg (27.3–32.6) and MCHC 245 g/l (316–349). Serum ferritin is 40 μg/l (15–200).

(iv) A 70-year-old Caucasian woman with rheumatoid arthritis has an FBC that shows RBC $3.10 \times 10^{12}/l$ (3.88–4.99), Hb 74 g/l (118–148), Hct 0.23 l/l (0.36–0.44), MCV 75.6 fl (82–98), MCH 23.8 pg (27.3–32.6) and MCHC 315 g/l l(316–349). Serum ferritin is 250 μg/l (15–200).

(v) A 74-year old Sudanese man has a routine blood count before surgery. It shows RBC $6.24 \times 10^{12}/l$ (4.32–5.66), Hb 141 g/l (133–167), Hct 0.45 l/l (0.39–0.50), MCV 72 fl (82–98), MCH 23 pg (27.3–32.6) and MCHC 313 g/l (316–349). Serum ferritin is 80 μg/l (15–200). Haemoglobin A_2 is 2.0% (2.5–3.5).

EMQ 9

For each clinical description of a patient with nodular lymphocyte-predominant Hodgkin lymphoma (NLPHL), select the most appropriate initial treatment from the alphabetical list. Each option can be used once, more than once or not at all.

a Alemtuzumab
b Combination chemotherapy
c Combination chemotherapy plus rituximab
d Involved field radiotherapy
e Involved field radiotherapy preceded by brief courses of combination chemotherapy
f Involved field radiotherapy with or without prior brief courses of combination chemotherapy
g ^{131}I tositumomab
h Mantle radiotherapy
i No further treatment indicated
j Rituximab monotherapy

   (i) A 32-year-old woman presents with left cervical lymphadenopathy. Biopsy of a cervical node shows NLPHL. She is asymptomatic and staging investigations show no evidence of other disease.

  (ii) A cervical lymph node completely excised from a 6-year-old boy shows NLPHL. He is asymptomatic. Staging investigations including positron emission tomography (PET)/CT scanning show no evidence of disease.

 (iii) A 33-year-old woman has right cervical and axillary lymphadenopathy and has lost 10% of body weight in the previous 6 months. Biopsy shows NLPHL.

 (iv) A 75-year old frail woman presents with cervical and inguinal lymphadenopathy and weight loss. Excision biopsy shows NLPHL.

  (v) A 48-year-old woman with a previous history of NLPHL treated by extended field radiotherapy presents with a mass of abdominal lymph nodes. Biopsy shows diffuse high grade B-cell lymphoma.

EMQ 10

For each clinical description of a patient with a cutaneous disorder, select the most likely diagnosis from the alphabetical list.

a Adult T-cell leukaemia/lymphoma
b Blastic plasmacytoid dendritic cell neoplasm
c Cutaneous mastocytosis
d Dermatitis herpetiformis
e Extramedullary plasmacytoma
f Myeloid sarcoma
g Neurofibromatosis
h Paraneoplastic pemphigus
i POEMS syndrome
j Systemic mastocytosis

(i) A 27-year-old woman presents with an intensely itchy raised red rash with groups of small blisters. She has an Hb of 97 g/l and an MCV of 105 fl. Skin biopsy shows granular IgA at the dermal–epidermal junction.

(ii) A 6-year-old girl presents with pallor and splenomegaly. She is noted to have multiple café-au-lait spots, freckles in her axillae and scoliosis. Her FBC shows anaemia, thrombocytopenia, leucocytosis and monocytosis.

(iii) A 62-year-old man presents with cutaneous nodules and plaques. A biopsy shows a monomorphic dermal infiltrate of medium-sized cells with delicate chromatin. There is some extension into subcutaneous fat. Immunohistochemistry shows expression of CD4, CD56 and CD123. There are occasional circulating agranular blast cells, some with blunt cytoplasmic tails.

(iv) A 58-year-old man presents with multiple pruritic hyperpigmented cutaneous lesions. He is found to have anaemia and leucopenia. Vigorous stroking of the cutaneous lesions leads to urtication.

(v) A 48-year-old woman presents with polyneuropathy, splenomegaly and skin thickening with hyperpigmentation and hypertrichosis. Further investigation shows her to have an IgG lambda paraprotein in a low concentration.

EMQ 11

For each clinical description select the most appropriate initial treatment from the alphabetical list.

a 3-product prothrombin concentrate
b 4-product prothrombin concentrate
c Cryoprecipitate
d Desmopressin plus tranexamic acid
e Either 3-product or 4-product prothrombin concentrate
f Factor V concentrate plus factor VIII concentrate
g Intermediate purity factor VIII concentrate
h Pathogen-inactivated fresh frozen plasma
i Pathogen-inactivated fresh frozen plasma plus supplementary factor VIII
j Tranexamic acid

    (i) A 38-year-old man with intramuscular bleeding resulting from combined factor V and factor VIII deficiency.

    (ii) A 23-year-old woman with factor XI deficiency with menorrhagia.

    (iii) A 32-year-old woman with significant bleeding resulting from factor X deficiency when specific product is not available.

    (iv) A 35-year-old man with significant bleeding from factor XIII deficiency when specific product is not available.

    (v) A 28-year-old man with type 1 von Willebrand disease who requires a dental extraction.

EMQ 12

For each clinicopathological description select the most likely diagnosis from the alphabetical list.

a Acute lymphoblastic leukaemia
b Burkitt lymphoma
c Chronic lymphocytic leukaemia
d Diffuse large B-cell lymphoma
e Follicular lymphoma
f Hairy cell leukaemia
g Mantle cell lymphoma
h Mucosa-associated lymphoid tissue (MALT) lymphoma
i Plasma cell leukaemia
j Splenic marginal zone lymphoma

(i)   A 60-year-old man has splenomegaly and pancytopenia with small numbers of abnormal circulating cells. These cells show high forward light scatter (FSC) and express CD11c, CD19, CD20 (strong), CD22 (strong), CD25, CD103, CD123, FMC7 and kappa-restricted strong surface membrane immunoglobulin (SmIg). There is no expression of CD5, CD23 or CD79b.

(ii) A 35-year-old man has generalised lymphadenopathy, anaemia and a high white cell count. His blood film shows lymphocytosis with medium-sized lymphoid cells with a fairly delicate chromatin pattern and basophilic cytoplasm with some cytoplasmic vacuoles. These cells express CD10, CD19, CD20, CD38, FMC7 and SmIg (lambda restricted). There is no expression of CD5, CD23 or TdT.

(iii) A 69-year-old man with lymphocytosis has no abnormal physical findings. His blood film shows small, apparently mature lymphocytes. Immunophenotyping shows expression of CD5, CD20 (weak), CD22 (very weak), CD23, CD38, CD200 and SmIg (weak, kappa restricted). There is no expression of CD79b or FMC7.

(iv) A 60-year-old man presents with renal failure and confusion. There are no specific findings on physical examination. A blood film shows medium-sized, pleomorphic lymphoid cells with moderately basophilic cytoplasm; some have nucleoli. Immunophenotyping shows expression of CD38 and CD56. There is no expression of CD5, CD19, CD20, CD22, CD23 or SmIg.

(v)   A 53-year-old woman presents with generalised lymphadenopathy and lymphocytosis. A blood film shows pleomorphic lymphoid cells, some of which are cleft and some nucleolated. Immunophenotyping shows expression of CD5, CD19, CD20, CD22, CD79b, FMC7 and moderately strong SmIg (kappa restricted). There is weak expression of CD23 and no expression of CD200.

EMQ 13

For each clinical description select from the alphabetical list the most appropriate initial treatment of the thrombocytopenia, in addition to avoidance of aspirin and non-steroidal anti-inflammatory drugs.

a Anti-D
b Corticosteroids
c High dose intravenous immunoglobulin
d No specific treatment
e Plasma exchange
f Platelet transfusion
g Platelet transfusion plus fresh frozen plasma/cryoprecipitate
h Rituximab
i Splenectomy
j Thrombopoietin receptor agonist

(i) An 8-year-old boy presents with bruising and is found to have scattered petechiae but no other detectable abnormality. His platelet count is $9 \times 10^9/l$. A blood film confirms the count and shows mainly normal-sized platelets.

(ii) A 6-year-old boy requiring minor surgery is found on routine preoperative testing to have a platelet count of $15 \times 10^9/l$. There is no history of bleeding. His blood film shows very large platelets and ill-defined cytoplasmic inclusions in neutrophils.

(iii) An 8-year-old boy who presents with oral bleeding and is found to have bruises, petechiae, oral blood blisters and bleeding from the mouth and pharynx. His platelet count is $9 \times 10^9/l$. A blood film confirms the count and shows mainly normal sized platelets.

(iv) A 10-year-old boy presents with pallor and fatigue. He is noted to have several bruises. His FBC shows WBC $7.4 \times 10^9/l$, Hb 90 g/l and platelet count $19 \times 10^9/l$. A blood film confirms the thrombocytopenia and shows immature granulated cells. Fibrinogen is 0.8 g/l. Following the venepuncture, he is noted to have bruised around the venepuncture site.

(v) An 8-year-old boy with type 1 diabetes mellitus and a previously normal platelet count presents with bruising and bleeding from his mouth. He has petechiae and bruising. His platelet count is $9 \times 10^9/l$. A blood film confirms the count and shows mainly normal sized platelets.

EMQ 14

For each clinicopathological description select the most likely diagnosis from the alphabetical list. Choose the most precise answer.

a Cold haemagglutinin disease (CHAD)
b Fanconi syndrome
c IgM myeloma
d Light chain associated amyloidosis
e Monoclonal gammopathy of undetermined significance (MGUS)
f Multiple myeloma (plasma cell myeloma)
g POEMS syndrome
h Type I cryoglobulinaemia
i Type II cryoglobulinaemia
j Waldenström macroglobulinaemia

   (i) A 71-year-old woman who is being investigated for a macro-cytic anaemia with normal serum B_{12} and folate assays is found to have an IgM paraprotein in a concentration of 11 g/l. No Bence–Jones protein is detected, skeletal survey is normal and bone marrow aspirate shows 8% plasma cells with dysplastic changes in 6% of erythroid cells.

   (ii) A 69-year-old woman presents with severe back pain and is found to have several crush fractures of vertebrae and lytic lesions in the skull. She is anaemic with an IgM paraprotein in a concentration of 32 g/l, reduced IgG and IgA and a kappa Bence–Jones protein in her urine. A bone marrow aspirate shows 15% clonal plasma cells, many of which are nucleolated.

   (iii) A 58-year-old woman presents with back pain. She is found to have hypouricaemia and glycosuria with a normal fasting glucose. FBC is normal. A bone marrow aspirate shows 2% plasma cells. Skeletal survey shows no lytic lesions but the patient is found to have osteomalacia.

   (iv) A 45-year-old man who is known to carry hepatitis C is noted to have a precipitate in his blood film. Investigation shows that he has a serum cryoglobulin, which is further characterised as composed of polyclonal IgG and monoclonal IgM.

   (v) A 58-year-old man presents with generalised lymphadenopathy and a sensorineural neuropathy. He has splenomegaly and skin pigmentation. Lymph node biopsy leads to a diagnosis of multicentric Castleman disease. Hb and WBC are normal; the platelet count is increased. Further investigation discloses a low concentration serum IgG lambda paraprotein and a bone marrow aspirate shows 5% plasma cells. Skeletal survey shows some osteosclerosis but no lytic lesions.

EMQ 15

For each pregnant woman being screened for relevant haemoglobinopathies and thalassaemia, select the most appropriate action from the list of options.

a No further action
b Perform DNA analysis for α^0 thalassaemia
c Perform sickle solubility test
d Prescribe iron and repeat analysis in a month
e Screen partner for α^0 thalassaemia
f Screen partner for β thalassaemia
g Screen partner for β thalassaemia and relevant haemoglobinopathies
h Screen partner for relevant haemoglobinopathies
i Test for an unstable haemoglobin
j Test patient and screen partner for α^0 thalassaemia

  (i)   An Italian woman whose FBC shows RBC 4.44×10^{12}/l, Hb 99 g/l, Hct 0.31 l/l, MCV 69 fl, MCH 22.3 pg and MCHC 319 g/l. Haemoglobin A_2 is 4.3%.
 (ii)   An Afro-Caribbean woman has normal red cell indices. Haemoglobin G Philadelphia is detected. Haemoglobin A_2 is 2.3%. Haemoglobin G_2 is also noted.
(iii)   The red cell indices of a Chinese woman are: RBC 5.78×10^{12}/l, Hb 105 g/l, Hct 0.32 l/l, MCV 56 fl, MCH 18.2 pg, MCHC 323 g/l. Haemoglobin A_2 is 3%.
 (iv)   The red cell indices of a Bangladeshi woman are RBC 4.22×10^{12}/l, Hb 70 g/l, Hct 0.29 l/l, MCV 67 fl, MCH 16.6 pg, MCHC 245 g/l. Hb A_2 is 3.4%.
  (v)   The red cell indices of an Afro-Caribbean woman are RBC 5.78×10^{12}/l, Hb 105 g/l, Hct 0.32 l/l, MCV 56 fl, MCH 18.2 pg, MCHC 323 g/l. Haemoglobin A_2 is 2.7%.

EMQ 16

For each clinical description select the most likely diagnosis from the alphabetical list.

a Autoimmune neutropenia
b Copper deficiency
c Cyclical neutropenia
d Drug-induced neutropenia
e Ethnic neutropenia
f Human immunodeficiency virus (HIV) infection
g Hypersplenism
h Myelodysplastic syndrome
i Vitamin B$_{12}$ deficiency
j Zinc deficiency

(i) A 30-year-old Greek woman with thalassaemia major is found to have a neutrophil count of 0.3×10^9/l. Her platelet count is normal and transfusion requirements have not altered.

(ii) A 75-year old Afro-Caribbean man presents with recurrent infection and is found to have a neutrophil count of 0.6×10^9/l, Hb of 120 g/l and MCV of 105 fl. Neutrophils are hypogranular and hypolobated.

(iii) A 60-year-old English man presents with recurrent infection and is found to have a palpable spleen. His neutrophil count is 0.8×10^9/l. His blood film shows increased numbers of large granular lymphocytes.

(iv) A 38-year-old, 100-kg English woman becomes neutropenic some time after bariatric surgery. The neutrophil count is 1.0×10^9/l.

(v) A 32-year-old Nigerian man presents with falciparum malaria. Following clearance of parasites he is found to have a neutrophil count persistently between 0.9 and 1.1×10^9/l.

EMQ 17

For each clinical description of a patient with cytopenia, select from the alphabetical list the gene that is most likely to be implicated.

a *DARC* (Duffy antigen receptor complex)
b *DKC1* (dyskerin)
c *ELANE* (neutrophil elastase)
d *FANCA* (*FANCA* gene)
e *LYST* (lysosomal trafficking regulator)
f *MYH9* (myosin heavy chain 9, non-muscle)
g *MYH11*(myosin heavy chain 11, non-muscle)
h *RPS19* (ribosomal subunit 19)
i *RUNX1* (runt-related transcription factor 1)
j *WAS* (Wiskott–Aldrich syndrome)

   (i) A 3-month-old Caucasian boy presents with pneumonia and is found to have a neutrophil count of 0.3 × 10^9/l, which does not improve. A bone marrow aspirate shows apparent arrest of granulopoiesis at the promyelocyte stage.

  (ii) A 20-year old Nigerian man is found to have a neutrophil count varying between 1 and 1.2 × 10^9/l.

 (iii) A 9-month-old Caucasian girl presents with listlessness and pallor. She is anaemic with an increased MCV and normal neutrophil and platelet counts. A bone marrow examination shows pure red cell aplasia.

 (iv) A 30-year-old man has an incidental finding of neutropenia. Serial counts show that the neutrophil count cycles with a periodicity of 2–3 weeks.

  (v) A 55-year-old presents with chronic kidney disease and sensorineural deafness. There is an incidental observation of thrombocytopenia (platelet count 80 × 10^9/l). His blood film shows large platelets and neutrophil inclusions.

EMQ 18

For each clinical description select the most appropriate diagnosis from the list of options.

a 5q– syndrome
b Autoimmune haemolytic anaemia
c Blackfan–Diamond syndrome
d Congenital dyserythropoietic anaemia
e Drug-induced macrocytosis
f Folic acid deficiency
g Refractory anaemia
h Refractory cytopenia with multilineage dysplasia
i Refractory cytopenia with ring sideroblasts
j Vitamin B_{12} deficiency

   (i) A 28-year-old man has a history of chronic diarrhoea and has previously had several episodes of unexplained iron deficiency anaemia. He presents with a macrocytic anaemia with hyper-segmented neutrophils.

   (ii) A 75-year-old woman with a previous history of hypothyroidism presents with anaemia and a peripheral neuropathy. Her blood film shows macrocytes, oval macrocytes and hypersegmented neutrophils. Assays show serum vitamin B_{12} of 170 ng/l (normal range 150–700) and serum folate of 10 µg/l (normal range 2–11). Lactate dehydrogenase is increased.

   (iii) A 32-year-old woman presents with pallor and fatigue and is found to have a macrocytic anaemia and an increased platelet count. Bone marrow examination shows a normocellular marrow with erythroid hypoplasia and hypolobated but normally sized megakaryocytes.

   (iv) A 72-year-old man with known chronic lymphocytic leukaemia presents with pallor and jaundice. His Hb is 85 g/l and MCV is 105 fl.

   (v) A 48-year-old woman who presents with fatigue is found to have an Hb of 78 g/l, an MCV of 110 fl and a platelet count of 503×10^9/l. Her blood film confirms macrocytosis and shows hypolobated, hypogranular neutrophils. Her bone marrow shows 17% ring sideroblasts. Blast cells are not increased.

EMQ 19

For each clinicopathological description select the most likely diagnosis from the alphabetical list.

a Adult T-cell leukaemia/lymphoma
b Blastic plasmacytoid dendritic cell neoplasm
c Dermatopathic lymphadenopathy
d Lymphoblastic lymphoma
e Mycosis fungoides
f Myeloid sarcoma
g Peripheral T-cell lymphoma, not otherwise specified
h Primary cutaneous follicle centre cell lymphoma
i Sézary syndrome
j T-prolymphocytic leukaemia

(i) A 65-year-old man presents with cutaneous patches, plaques and several fungating cutaneous tumours. Several of the lesions are ulcerated. His skin abnormalities first started several years previously. Blood count and film are normal. Histology shows band-like infiltrates of CD4-positive T cells and histiocytes in the dermis.

(ii) A 75-year-old man presents with erythroderma, pruritus, hair loss and generalised lymphadenopathy with nodes measuring up to 1.5 cm. His symptoms date back several months. His blood film shows 7% lymphocytes with irregularly lobulated nuclei. Immunophenotyping shows these cells to be CD2+, CD3+, CD4+ and CD5+. A skin biopsy shows intra-epidermal lymphoid accumulations.

(iii) A 45-year-old man with chronic myelogenous leukaemia being treated with imatinib presents with a subcutaneous mass. An aspirate of the mass shows medium sized cells with a high nucleocytoplasmic ratio, an immature chromatin pattern and cytoplasmic granules. A bone marrow aspirate is essentially normal.

(iv) A 50-year-old man presents with a splenomegaly, bilateral pleural effusions and skin infiltration. Skin biopsy shows dermal infiltration, particularly in a perivascular distribution. There is no epidermotropism. The patient has a lymphocytosis and circulating cells express CD3 (weak), CD4, CD7 and CD8.

(v) A 45-year-old Afro-Caribbean man presents with generalised lymphadenopathy, skin infiltration, hypercalcaemia and lymphocytosis. A skin biopsy shows Pautrier's microabscesses and perivascular dermal infiltration by CD4-positive T cells. A blood film shows pleomorphic lymphoid cells, many with lobulated nuclei.

EMQ 20

For each clinicopathological description, select the most likely diagnosis from the alphabetical list.

a α^0 thalassaemia heterozygosity
b α^+ thalassaemia heterozygosity
c β thalassaemia heterozygosity
d $\epsilon\gamma\delta\beta$ thalassaemia heterozygosity
e $\delta\beta$ thalassaemia heterozygosity
f Haemoglobin Bart's hydrops fetalis
g Haemoglobin E/β thalassaemia compound heterozygosity
h Haemoglobin E heterozygosity
i Haemoglobin H disease
j Hereditary persistence of fetal haemoglobin

(i)   An Arab woman's blood count shows Hb 85 g/l, MCV 56 fl and MCH 17.1 pg. High performance liquid chromatography (HPLC) shows haemoglobin A 86.5%, haemoglobin H 10.4%, haemoglobin F 1.6% and haemoglobin A_2 1.4%.

(ii) A Taiwanese man's blood count shows RBC 6.28 × 10^{12}/l, Hb 137 g/l, Hct 0.43 l/l, MCV 69.1 fl, MCH 21.7 pg and MCHC 316 g/l. HPLC shows 1% haemoglobin F and 2.2% haemoglobin A_2.

(iii) A West African woman's blood count shows RBC 3.97 × 10^{12}/l, Hb 117 g/l, Hct 0.34 l/l, MCV 87 fl, MCH 29.4 pg and MCHC 343 g/l. HPLC shows 20% haemoglobin F and 1.8% haemoglobin A_2.

(iv) A Sri Lankan woman's blood count shows RBC 4.39 × 10^{12}/l, Hb 110 g/l, Hct 0.32 l/l, MCV 74 fl, MCH 25.1 pg and MCHC 332 g/l. HPLC shows 28% of haemoglobin to be in the A_2 window.

(v)   A 38-year-old African man's blood count shows RBC 5.97 × 10^{12}/l, Hb 130 g/l, Hct 0.38 l/l, MCV 64.2 fl, MCH 21.8 pg and MCHC 342 g/l. HPLC shows 3.0% haemoglobin F and 9.2% haemoglobin A_2.

EMQ 21

For each clinical description select the most likely diagnosis from the alphabetical list.

a Congenital amegakaryocytic thrombocytopenia with radio-ulnar synostosis
b Congenital parvovirus B19 infection
c Congenital rubella infection
d Diamond–Blackfan anaemia
e Dyskeratosis congenita
f Familial platelet disorder with propensity to myeloid malignancy
g Fanconi anaemia
h *MYH9*-related disorder
i Shwachman–Diamond syndrome
j Thrombocytopenia with absent radii

    (i) A 10-year-old boy presents with pancytopenia and is found to have a hypoplastic bone marrow. He is noted to have absent thumbs and café-au-lait spots. A sibling has microcephaly. Investigations show increased chromosomal breakage on exposure to diepoxybutane.

    (ii) A 3-month-old baby with a cleft palate is found to have a macrocytic anaemia with a low reticulocyte count and normal white cell and platelet counts. A bone marrow aspirate shows pure red cell aplasia. Red cell adenosine deaminase and the percentage of haemoglobin F are found to be elevated.

    (iii) An 8-year-old, abnormally short boy presents with steatorrhoea and is found to have neutropenia.

    (iv) A newborn baby is noted to have micrognathia, low set ears and a deformity of the arms and hands but with both thumbs being present. X-rays show absent radii. There is thrombocytopenia with normal-sized platelets.

    (v) A 10-year-old boy presents with pancytopenia and is found to have a hypocellular bone marrow. He is noted to have oral leukoplakia, dystrophic nails and a mottled appearance of the skin.

EMQ 22

For each clinicopathological description select the most likely diagnosis from the alphabetical list.

a α^0 thalassaemia heterozygosity
b α^+ thalassaemia heterozygosity
c β thalassaemia heterozygosity
d $\delta\beta$ thalassaemia
e Acaeruloplasminaemia
f Congenital sideroblastic anaemia
g Hereditary persistence of fetal haemoglobin
h Hypotransferrinaemia
i Iron-refractory iron deficiency anaemia
j Pearson syndrome

   (i) A 38-year-old Caucasian man presents with extrapyramidal and cerebellar symptoms and signs and is found to have retinal degeneration. He has a mild anaemia with mild microcytosis, low serum iron, normal transferrin, low transferrin saturation and elevated serum ferritin. He subsequently develops diabetes mellitus.

  (ii) A 5-year-old Caucasian boy presents with failure to thrive, hypochromic microcytic anaemia, low serum iron and very low, fully saturated transferrin.

 (iii) A 32-year-old pregnant Spanish woman is found on routine screening to have hypochromia and microcytosis without anaemia. Her serum ferritin is normal. High performance liquid chromatography shows haemoglobin A_2 of 2.5% and haemoglobin F of 11%. Distribution of haemoglobin F is heterogeneous.

 (iv) A 7-year-old boy Caucasian is found to have an MCV of 67 fl with an Hb of 113 g/l. His blood film shows microcytosis and mild poikilocytosis with no definite dimorphism. Serum ferritin is not reduced and haemoglobin A_2 percentage is normal. His mother is found to have an Hb of 107 g/l and a clearly dimorphic film. Her serum ferritin is elevated.

  (v) A 28-year-old pregnant Chinese woman is found on routine screening to have an Hb of 118 g/l and an MCH of 26 pg. Her blood film shows microcytosis and mild hypochromia. High performance liquid chromatography shows a haemoglobin A_2 of 2%.

EMQ 23

For each patient described select the most appropriate treatment from the alphabetical list.

a Corticosteroids
b Drug withdrawal
c Drug withdrawal plus rituximab
d Eculizumab
e Eculizumab followed by immunosuppression
f Eculizumab preceded by plasma infusion or exchange
g Haemodialysis
h Plasma exchange
i Plasma exchange plus corticosteroids
j Plasma infusion plus corticosteroids

(i) A 68-year-old woman with carcinoma of the pancreas and previous splenectomy is receiving gemcitabine. She is also receiving opiate analgesics for abdominal pain. Following a course of gemcitabine she is found to have a microangiopathic haemolytic anaemia with thrombocytopenia and an increased creatinine.

(ii) A 33-year-old woman develops hypertension and thrombotic microangiopathy and is found to have a deficiency of complement factor H.

(iii) A 10-year-old boy develops severe abdominal pain and bloody diarrhoea followed by acute kidney injury and a microangiopathic haemolytic anaemia following a farm visit. He has oliguria, fluid retention and a creatinine of 200 μmol/l.

(iv) A 38-year-old woman presents with fever and confusion and is found to have microangiopathic haemolytic anaemia, thrombocytopenia and a creatinine of 150 μmol/l. An ADAMTS13 assay has been requested.

(v) A 48-year-old woman presents with thrombotic microangiopathy and elevated creatinine. She has a normal level of ADAMTS13. Complement factor H is reduced and she is found to have antibodies to factor H.

EMQ 24

For each clinical description select the most likely cytogenetic abnormality from the alphabetical list.

a t(1;19)(q23;p13.3)
b t(2;5)(p23;q35)
c t(4;11)(q21;q23)
d t(5;14)(q31;q32)
e t(8;14)(q24;q32)
f t(9;22)(q34;q11.2)
g t(10;11)(p13;q14)
h t(11;14)(q13;q32)
i t(12;21)(p13;q22)
j t(14;18)(q32;q21)

(i) A 10-year-old girl presents with pallor and lymphadenopathy. A peripheral blood film shows blast cells. Immunophenotyping shows expression of CD10, CD13, CD19, CD34 and TdT. Other myeloid markers and SmIg are negative.

(ii) A 40-year-old HIV-positive man presents with lymphadenopathy. A peripheral blood film shows medium-sized lymphoid cells with cytoplasmic vacuolation. Immunophenotyping shows expression of CD20, CD19, CD79b, FMC7 and SmIg (kappa). There is no expression of CD5 or TdT.

(iii) A 60-year-old woman who presents with minor symptoms is discovered to have splenomegaly (spleen 4 cm below the left costal margin) and generalised lymphadenopathy (nodes 1–2 cm). A blood film shows small lymphoid cells with dense chromatin. Some have nuclear notches or clefts. Immunophenotyping shows expression of CD10, CD19, CD20, CD79b, FMC7 and SmIg (lambda). There is no expression of CD5, CD34 or TdT.

(iv) A 70-year-old woman presents with fatigue and weight loss. She is found to have generalised lymphadenopathy with nodes up to 2–3 cm in diameter. A peripheral blood film shows pleomorphic medium-sized lymphoid cells, some with nucleoli and some with irregular or cleft nuclei. Immunophenotyping shows expression of CD5, CD19, CD20, CD79b, FMC7 and SmIg (lambda). There is weak partial expression of CD23.

(v) An 80-year-old woman presents with pallor and lymphad-enopathy. A peripheral blood film shows blast cells. Immu-nophenotyping shows expression of CD10, CD13, CD19, CD25, CD33 and TdT. There is no expression of CD34 or SmIg.

EMQ 25

For each clinical description select the most likely diagnosis from the alphabetical list.

a Allergic bronchopulmonary aspergillosis
b Aspergilloma
c Chronic eosinophilic leukaemia, not otherwise specified
d Eosinophilic granulomatosis with polyangiitis
e Hodgkin lymphoma
f Idiopathic hypereosinophilic syndrome
g Myeloid neoplasm with rearrangement of *PDGFRA*
h Myeloid neoplasm with rearrangement of *PDGFRB*
i Parasitic infection
j Systemic mastocytosis

(i) A 38-year-old woman with a history of hay fever and adult onset asthma presents to a neurologist who finds her to have mononeuritis multiplex. Her eosinophil count is $1.7 \times 10^9/l$ (13%). She is found to have perinuclear antineutrophil cytoplasmic antibodies (p-ANCA). ESR and C-reactive protein (CRP) are increased. Chest X-ray shows ill-defined interstitial infiltrates.

(ii) A 35-year-old man has cervical lymphadenopathy and weight loss. He gives a history of alcohol-induced chest pain. His blood count shows WBC $12.4 \times 10^9/l$, Hb 113 g/l, MCV 78 fl, neutrophil count $7.2 \times 10^9/l$, eosinophil count $2.3 \times 10^9/l$ and platelet count $450 \times 10^9/l$. Chest X-ray shows left hilar lymphadenopathy. ESR is 48 mm in 1 h.

(iii) A 32-year-old man presents with worsening asthma, cough, fever, expectoration of mucus plugs and recent haemoptysis. Blood tests show an eosinophil count of $3.3 \times 10^9/l$. Serum IgE is increased. p-ANCA antibodies are not detected. Chest X-ray shows infiltrates in the middle and upper lobes and proximal bronchiectasis.

(iv) A 35-year-old North African man presents with a history of intermittent haematuria and is found to have a normocytic normochromic anaemia and eosinophilia.

(v) A 42-year-old man presents with a rash and breathlessness. He is found to have a cardiac murmur and mild heart failure. FBC shows an eosinophil count of $3.4 \times 10^9/l$. Serum tryptase is mildly elevated. A bone marrow aspirate and trephine biopsy show increased eosinophils and precursors and the trephine biopsy also shows increased interstitial mast cells. Fluorescence *in situ* hybridisation (FISH) shows deletion of the *CHIC2* gene.

EMQ 26

For each clinical description select the most appropriate diagnosis from the list of options.

a Chronic cold haemagglutinin disease
b Delayed haemolytic transfusion reaction
c Epstein–Barr virus-related cold antibody-mediated haemolysis
d Glucose-6-phosphate dehydrogenase (G6PD) deficiency
e Megaloblastic anaemia
f *Mycoplasma pneumoniae*-related cold antibody-mediated haemolysis.
g Paroxysmal cold haemoglobinuria (PCH)
h Paroxysmal nocturnal haemoglobinuria (PNH)
i Unstable haemoglobin
j Warm autoimmune haemolytic anaemia

(i) A 4-year-old girl presents with pallor and jaundice. She has recently suffered an upper respiratory tract infection. Her Hb is 80 g/l and reticulocyte count $50 \times 10^9/l$. Her blood film shows spherocytes, red cell agglutinates and erythrophagocytosis by neutrophils. A direct antiglobulin test (DAT) detects C3 but not immunoglobulin (Ig).

(ii) A 75-year-old man presents with jaundice and pallor two weeks after surgery for a ruptured abdominal aortic aneurysm. He is found to have an Hb of 92 g/l and a positive DAT for IgG and complement. Microscopy shows mixed field agglutination.

(iii) A 10-year-old girl presents with a history of intermittent jaundice and passing of dark urine. Her spleen is palpable 3 cm below the left costal margin. Her father has had similar episodes all his life. She has recovered from a recent episode and her FBC now shows WBC $7.8 \times 10^9/l$, Hb 110 g/l, MCV 102 fl, MCHC 294 g/l and platelet count $98 \times 10^9/l$. Her blood film shows small numbers of irregularly contracted cells and macrocytes. Bilirubin and lactate dehydrogenase (LDH) are mildly elevated.

(iv) A 75-year-old man presents with acrocyanosis and a history of intermittently passing dark urine. An automated full blood count shows WBC $7.6 \times 10^9/l$, lymphocytes $4.3 \times 10^9/l$, Hb 65 g/l, MCV 125 fl and platelets $144 \times 10^9/l$.

(v) A 17-year-old student presents with symptomatic anaemia and jaundice. He gives a history that 2 weeks previously he had developed fever, a sore throat and swelling of his neck but he had not sought medical attention. His Hb is 62 g/l and reticulocyte count $210 \times 10^9/l$. A blood film shows red cell agglutinates, polychromasia and atypical lymphocytes. Serology shows a high titre cold agglutinin with anti-i specificity.

EMQ 27

For each clinical description, select the most likely explanation for the measured haemoglobin concentration from the list options.

a Chronic renal failure
b Delayed haemolytic transfusion reaction
c Folic acid deficiency
d Hyperhaemolysis
e Hypersplenism
f Iron deficiency
g Normal for this patient
h Parvovirus B19 infection
i Splenic infarction
j Splenic sequestration

(i) A 44-year-old man with sickle cell/haemoglobin C disease has had a slow decline of his Hb over the previous 3 years. His Hb in now 50 g/l and his MCV 81 fl.

(ii) A 21-year-old woman with sickle cell anaemia has an Hb of 75 g/l at a routine clinic visit. MCV is 85 fl. She has recently had an upper respiratory tract infection.

(iii) A 2-year-old girl with sickle cell anaemia presents with acute anaemia. Her Hb is 35 g/l. Her spleen is palpable at the level of the umbilicus.

(iv) A 7-year-old girl with sickle cell anaemia presents with an Hb of 40 g/l and a reticulocyte count of 5 × 10⁹/l. She appears listless.

(v) A 20-year-old man with sickle cell anaemia presents in chest crisis with an Hb of 80 g/l. He is transfused two units of ABO-compatible Kell-negative packed red cells. 72 hours later he has tachycardia and jaundice. His Hb is found to be 55 g/l.

EMQ 28

For each clinicopathological description select the most likely cytogenetic abnormality from the alphabetical list.

a inv(3)(q21q26)
b inv(16)(p13.1q22)
c t(1;22)(p13;q13)
d t(5;12)(q31-33;p12)
e t(6;9)(p23;q34)
f t(8;21)(q22;q22)
g t(9;11)(p22;q23)
h t(9;22)(q34;q11.2)
i t(12;21)(q13)(q22)
j t(15;17)(q22;q12)

(i) A 2-year-old child presents with marked hepatosplenomegaly with 25% bone marrow blast cells and bone marrow fibrosis. Immunophenotyping shows the blast cells to be megakaryo-blasts.

(ii) A 58-year-old woman presents with symptoms of anaemia and is found to have splenomegaly and a minor degree of hepatomegaly. Her FBC shows WBC 23 × 10⁹/l, neutrophils 70%, lymphocytes 9%, eosinophils 10% (2.3 × 10⁹/l), monocytes 9% (2.1 × 10⁹/l), basophils 0%, myelocytes 1% and blast cells 1%.

(iii) A 25-year-old man presents with symptoms of anaemia and bruising. His FBC shows pancytopenia with small numbers of blast cells. Bone marrow examination shows trilineage dysplasia and 60% blast cells with both neutrophilic and basophilic differentiation.

(iv) A 24-year-old man presents with epistaxis and bruising. There is no organomegaly. His full blood count shows WBC $23 \times 10^9/l$, Hb 125 g/l and platelet count $30 \times 10^9/l$. The majority of circulating white cells are bilobed cells, some with very fine azurophilic granules.

(v) A 40-year-old woman presents with fatigue. Her FBC shows WBC $27 \times 10^9/l$, Hb 81 g/l and platelet count $80 \times 10^9/l$. A blood film shows blast cells, increased monocytes and pro-monocytes and increased eosinophils, which are mainly cytologically normal. Bone marrow examination shows that blast cells (cytologically both myeloblasts and monoblasts) plus promonocytes constitute 80% of bone marrow cells. There are 10% of cells of eosinophil lineage including eosinophil precursors with large purple granules. Some Charcot–Leyden crystals are seen.

EMQ 29

For each clinical description of a patient with an infection, select the most likely mechanism of haemolysis from the alphabetical list.

a Arrest of erythropoiesis
b Erythrocyte membrane damage by exotoxin
c Haemolysis due to a cold agglutinin with anti-i specificity
d Haemolysis due to a cold agglutinin with anti-I specificity
e Haemolysis due to anti-P antibody
f Haemolysis due to invasion of erythrocytes
g Haemolysis due to invasion and rosetting of erythrocytes
h Haemophagocytic lymphohistiocytosis
i Microangiopathic haemolytic anaemia
j T activation

(i) A young man with *Plasmodium falciparum* malaria has an Hb of 110 g/l and a reticulocyte count of 200 × 10^9/l.

(ii) A 7-year-old girl with hereditary spherocytosis whose Hb is usually 90–100 g/l presents with an Hb of 60 g/l and a reticulocyte count of 5 × 10^9/l following a febrile illness with a rash.

(iii) A 5-year-old boy presents with jaundice following an episode of diarrhoea and is found to have an Hb of 62 g/l and a reticulocyte count of 234 × 10^9/l. His serum creatinine is increased.

(iv) A 23-year-old woman has an illegal abortion in a country where legal termination of pregnancy is difficult. She develops fever and jaundice and appears very unwell. Her Hb is 67 g/l. A blood film shows spherocytosis and polychromasia.

(v) A 28-year-old woman develops fever and a cough and chest radiography shows patchy consolidation. She becomes anaemic and her blood film shown red cell agglutinates.

EMQ 30

For each clinicopathological description select the most likely diagnosis from the list of options.

a Atypical haemolytic uraemic syndrome
b Dehydrated hereditary stomatocytosis (xerocytosis)
c Glucose-6-phophate dehydrogenase (G6PD) deficiency
d Haemoglobin Köln heterozygosity
e Hereditary pyropoikilocytosis
f Overhydrated hereditary stomatocytosis
g Phytosterolaemia
h Pyrimidine 5' nucleotidase deficiency
i Pyruvate kinase deficiency
j South-east Asian ovalocytosis

(i) A 25-year-old woman being investigated as part of a family study is found to have a mild haemolytic anaemia and thrombocytopenia with her blood film showing numerous stomatocytes and very large platelets.

(ii) A 6-year-old girl with pallor and splenomegaly is found to have a moderately severe haemolytic anaemia. Her blood film shows marked poikilocytosis including some elliptocytes. Her father's blood film shows elliptocytes while her mother's film is normal. Eosin-5-maleimide binding is found to be reduced.

(iii) A 16-year-old girl has had a splenectomy because of a chronic haemolytic anaemia. She subsequently suffers recurrent episodes of venous thromboembolism. Her blood film shows post-splenectomy changes, including marked thrombocytosis, and also numerous stomatocytes.

(iv) A 12-year-old girl with a past history of neonatal jaundice has a moderately severe haemolytic anaemia. Her blood film shows prominent basophilic stippling.

(v) A 24-year-old man of Sicilian ancestry presents with acute haemolysis following a febrile illness. His blood film shows irregularly contracted cells.

Section 4:
Single Best Answers
Answers to Questions 1–120
with Feedback

Multiple Choice Questions for Haematology and Core Medical Trainees, First Edition.
Barbara J. Bain.
© 2016 John Wiley & Sons, Ltd. Published 2016 by John Wiley & Sons, Ltd.

SBA 1 b Chronic lymphocytic leukaemia.

The features described are typical of this condition and this is often an incidental diagnosis in a patient presenting with another condition. Smear cells are typical of chronic lymphocytic leukaemia, but not pathognomonic; they are indicative of the fragility of the cells, which causes them to be disrupted when the film is spread. In view of the patient's ethnic origin, a diagnosis of adult T-cell leukaemia/lymphoma should also be considered but the typical blood film features (lymphocytes with lobulated and flower-shaped nuclei) are missing; in addition this lymphoma is usually aggressive and is thus much less likely to be an incidental diagnosis.

SBA 2 c JC virus.

The features described suggest a diagnosis of progressive multifocal leucoencephalopathy, which is caused by this virus.[1] The underlying cause is immune deficiency including the acquired immune deficiency syndrome (AIDS), chemotherapy (particularly for B-cell lymphoma and leukaemia), immunosuppressive therapy such as mycophenolate mofetil following organ transplantation and monoclonal antibody therapy (including rituximab for lymphoma/leukaemia, natalizumab for multiple sclerosis or Crohn disease, efalizumab for psoriasis and infliximab for multiple conditions). Efalizumab has now been withdrawn from the market because of this risk.

Reference

1. Ferenczy MV, Marshall LJ, Nelson CD, Atwood WJ, Nath A, Khalili K and Major EO (2012) Molecular biology, epidemiology, and pathogenesis of progressive multifocal leukoencephalopathy, the JC virus-induced demyelinating disease of the human brain. *Clin Microbiol Rev*, 25, 471–507. PMID: 22763635

SBA 3 b 70 g/l.

Numerous trials of patients in different circumstances have shown the benefits of a restrictive rather than a liberal transfusion policy. A transfusion threshold of 70 g/l has been found equivalent to or no worse than a more liberal transfusion policy. With regard to sepsis, no benefit has been found with a higher transfusion threshold.[1,2]

References

1. Holst LB, Haase N, Wetterslev J, Wernerman J, Guttormsen AB, Karlsson S *et al*. TRISS Trial Group; Scandinavian Critical Care Trials Group (2014) Lower versus higher hemoglobin threshold for transfusion in septic shock. *N Engl J Med*, 371, 1381–1391. PMID:25270275
2. Hébert PC and Carson JL (2014) Transfusion threshold of 7 g per deciliter—the new normal. *N Engl J Med*, 371, 1459–1461. PMID: 25270276

SBA 4 c Haematological features of anorexia nervosa.

The haematological abnormalities are all attributable to anorexia nervosa *per se* and can be related to bone marrow hypocellularity and gelatinous transformation.[1]

Reference

1. Sabel AL, Gaudiani JL, Statland B and Mehler PS (2013) Hematological abnormalities in severe anorexia nervosa. *Ann Hematol*, 92, 605–613. PMID: 23392575

SBA 5 c Anaemia of chronic disease plus iron deficiency.

Both iron deficiency and severe anaemia of chronic disease can cause a microcytic anaemia with reduction of serum iron and transferrin concentration.[1] Interpretation of the blood count and biochemical measurements together suggests that the patient has both iron deficiency and anaemia of chronic disease. There are clear signs of active inflammation in the elevated erythrocyte sedimentation rate (ESR), rouleaux formation, WBC and neutrophil count. This would be expected to cause an increase in serum ferritin and a reduction of the iron binding capacity. Uncomplicated iron deficiency is associated with a serum ferritin of less than 14 µg/l but in the presence of inflammation values up to 50 or even 100 µg/l can be seen. The relatively high total iron binding capacity for a patient with acute inflammation also points in the direction of iron deficiency. α and β thalassaemia trait would be expected to cause microcytosis without significant anaemia.

Reference

1. DeLoughery TG (2014) Microcytic anemia. *N Engl J Med*, 371, 1324–1331. PMID: 25271605

SBA 6 a Lead poisoning.

The clinical and laboratory features are those of lead poisoning.[1-5] The patient had been working for some months, stripping paint and redecorating an old house. In assessing a patient with suspected lead poisoning it is also important to be aware that Ayurvedic medicines may contain lead. Even in the UK, drinking water sometimes has toxic levels of lead.[6]

References

1. Frith D, Yeung K, Thrush S, Hunt BJ and Hubbard JG (2005) Lead poisoning—a differential diagnosis for abdominal pain. *Lancet*, 366, 2146. PMID: 16360796
2. Pol RR and Howard MR (2014) A man with anemia and a change in personality. *Blood*, 123, 1784. PMID: 24783257
3. Friedman LS, Simmons LH, Goldman RH and Sohani AR (2014) Case records of the Massachusetts General Hospital. Case 12-2014. A 59-year-old man with fatigue, abdominal pain, anemia, and abnormal liver function. *N Engl J Med*, 370, 1542–1550. PMID: 24738672
4. Kathuria P (2014) Lead toxicity. http://emedicine.medscape.com/article/1174752-overview (accessed June 2015)
5. Health and Safety Executive, Exposure to lead. http://www.hse.gov.uk/STATISTICS/causdis/lead/index.htm (accessed June 2015)
6. Pickrell WO, Hirst C, Brunt H and Pearson OR (2013) Peripheral neuropathy—lead astray. *Lancet*, 381, 1156. PMID: 23540854

SBA 7 d Plegmasia caerulea dolens.

Plegmasia caerulea dolens results from extensive deep vein thrombosis with complete obstruction of deep and superficial veins, this in turn often leading to arterial insufficiency.[1,2] In plegmasia alba dolens, on the other hand, some drainage through superficial veins is retained. The severe unilateral oedema would not occur in a primarily arterial problem. The extensive thrombosis despite warfarin therapy suggests a hypercoagulable state and in this age range underlying carcinoma could be suspected.

References

1. Dradik A and Liem T (2014) Phlegmasia alba and cerulea dolens. http://emedicine.medscape.com/article/461809-overview (accessed June 2015)
2. Gibson CJ, Britton KA, Miller AL and Lascalzo J (2014) Out of the blue. *N Engl J Med*, 270, 1742–1748. PMID: 24785210

SBA 8 e Ig (immunoglobulin) A anti-tissue transglutaminase antibodies.

The clinical history suggests coeliac disease.[1] The recommended first line test (National Institute for Health and Care Excellence (NICE) guidelines) is IgA anti-tissue transglutaminase antibodies. If this is negative, IgA should be assayed and, in deficient patients (2% of those with coeliac disease), tests for IgG anti-tissue transglutaminase and antiendomysial antibodies should be done.[2] About 5% of patients with coeliac disease do not have antibodies to tissue transglutaminase.[3] Diagnosis then depends on antibodies to endomysium or to deamidated gliadin peptide.[3] It is important that patients continue on a gluten-containing diet until serological evaluation and duodenal biopsy are done.

References

1. Mooney PD, Hadjivassiliou M and Sanders DS (2014) Coeliac disease. *BMJ*, 348, 30–34. PMID: 24589518
2. Richey R, Howdle P, Shaw E and Stokes T on behalf of the Guideline Development Group (2009) Recognition and assessment of coeliac disease in children and adults: summary of NICE guidance. *BMJ*, 38, 1386–1387. PMID:19474030
3. Leffler D (2011) Celiac disease diagnosis and management: a 46-year-old woman with anemia. *JAMA*, 306, 1582–1592. PMID: 21990301

SBA 9 e Human immunodeficiency virus.

Escherichia coli O157:H7 is the usual cause of haemolytic uraemic syndrome while *Escherichia coli* O104:H4 was responsible for a German outbreak of this syndrome in 2011. However this patient has features suggesting a diagnosis of thrombotic thrombocytopenic purpura (TTP).[1,2] It is important that all patients presenting with TTP are tested for human immunodeficiency virus (HIV) since TTP may be the presenting feature of HIV infection. Some patients with HIV infection and TTP have a low ADAMTS13 and an ADAMTS13 antibody whereas others do not have an ADAMTS13 deficiency. Those who are deficient require plasma exchange as well as highly active anti-retroviral therapy.

References

1. Hunt BJ (2014) Bleeding and coagulopathies in critical care. *N Engl J Med*, 370, 2153. PMID: 24869733

2. Scully M, Hunt BJ, Benjamin S, Liesner R, Rose P, Peyvandi F *et al.*; British Committee for Standards in Haematology (2012) Guidelines on the diagnosis and management of thrombotic thrombocytopenic purpura and other thrombotic microangiopathies. *Br J Haematol,* 158, 323–335. PMID: 22624596

SBA 10 b Hepatitis B.

The infection most readily transmitted by needle prick injury is hepatitis B with reported transmission rates of 7–30%, followed by hepatitis C (reported rates 0–7%) then HIV (about 0.5%). Occasional examples of transmission of dengue fever have been reported.

Reference

Bain BJ. *Blood Cells,* 5th Edn, Wiley-Blackwell, Oxford, 2015.

SBA 11 d Hereditary haemorrhagic telangiectasia.

The patient appears to have iron deficiency anaemia and has telangiectasia and a pulmonary arteriovenous malformation. This constellation of abnormalities suggests hereditary haemorrhagic telangiectasia.[1] The chronic iron deficiency anaemia is the result of chronic blood loss from intestinal telangiectasia. Heyde syndrome is acquired von Willebrand disease due to sheer stress due in turn to vascular lesions such as aortic stenosis;[2] it is not associated with pulmonary arteriovenous malformations. The patient does not have the other clinical features of CREST.

Diagnostic criteria suggested for hereditary haemorrhagic telangiectasia are that the patient should have at least three out of four of (i) epistaxis; (ii) telangiectasia (typically affecting lips, mouth, fingers or nose); (iii) visceral lesions (such as gastrointestinal telangiectasia or arteriovenous malformations in the lung, liver, brain or spinal cord) and (iv) an appropriate family history.[3]

Hereditary haemorrhagic telangiectasia is of relevance to haematologists and physicians as a cause of chronic iron deficiency anaemia. There is also an increased prevalence of venous thromboembolism, possibly as a result of an increased concentration of factor VIII.

References

1. Salaria M, Taylor J, Bogwitz M and Winship I (2014) Hereditary haemorrhagic telangiectasia, an Australian cohort: clinical and investigative features. *Intern Med J*, 44, 639–644. PMID: 24750312
2. Sadler JE (2003) Aortic stenosis, von Willebrand factor, and bleeding. *N Engl J Med*, 349, 323–325. PMID: 12878737
3. Shovlin CL, Guttmacher AE, Buscarini E, Faughnan ME, Hyland RH, Westermann CJ *et al.* (2000) Diagnostic criteria for hereditary hemorrhagic telangiectasia (Rendu-Osler-Weber syndrome). *Am J Med Genet*, 91, 66–67. PMID: 10751092

SBA 12 e *Streptococcus pneumonia.*

There is an increased risk of infection by all these organisms following splenectomy but the most likely in this patient is *Streptococcus pneumonia.*[1]

Reference

1. Rubin LG and Schaffner W (2014) Care of the asplenic patient. *N Engl J Med*, 371, 349–356. PMID: 25054718

SBA 13 e Sinusoidal obstruction syndrome.

The features described suggest sinusoidal obstruction syndrome, previously known as hepatic veno-occlusive disease.[1,2] Damage to hepatic endothelial cells by the preparatory regime, particularly busulphan and total body irradiation, results in deposition of fibrin in hepatic sinusoids and congestion by erythrocytes; centrilobular hepatic necrosis can occur, followed by fibrous obliteration and occlusion of terminal venules. Hepatic failure and death can result.

References

1. Dignan FL, Wynn RF, Hadzic N, Karani J, Quaglia A, Pagliuca A *et al.*; Haemato-oncology Task Force of British Committee for Standards in Haematology; British Society for Blood and Marrow Transplantation (2013) BCSH/BSBMT guideline: diagnosis and management of veno-occlusive disease (sinusoidal obstruction syndrome) following haematopoietic stem cell transplantation. *Br J Haematol*, 163, 444–457. PMID: 24102514
2. Chao N (2014) How I treat sinusoidal obstruction syndrome. *Blood*, 123, 4023–4026. PMID: 24833355

SBA 14 b Acute myeloid leukaemia, breast cancer, hypothyroidism and coronary artery disease.

The patient has an increased risk of hypothyroidism and breast cancer as a result of the mantle radiotherapy and an increased risk of acute myeloid leukaemia as a result of the chemotherapy (doxorubicin).[1,2] There is a slight increase in the risk of acute lymphoblastic leukaemia following the use of topoisomerase-interactive drugs such as doxorubicin but b is a better answer than a as the risk of hypothyroidism and breast cancer is quite high. Bladder cancer is increased after cyclophosphamide and ifosfamide but the patient did not receive these drugs.

The patient should be having an annual mammogram and monitoring of thyroid function is also indicated.

References

1. Suh E, Daugherty CK, Wroblewski K, Lee H, Kigin ML, Rasinski KA et al. (2014) General internists' preferences and knowledge about the care of adult survivors of childhood cancer: a cross-sectional survey. Ann Intern Med, 160, 11–17. PMID: 24573662
2. Children's Oncology Group. Long-term follow-up guidelines for survivors of childhood, adolescent and young adult cancers, Version 3.0. Arcadia, CA: Children's Oncology Group; October 2008; Available on-line: www.survivorshipguidelines.org (accessed June 2015)

SBA 15 c She should take supplementary folic acid.

If the patient's coeliac disease has responded well to a gluten-free diet her absorption of iron, folic acid and vitamin B_{12} may now be normal. However all pregnant women are advised to take 0.4 mg daily of folic acid from before conception to 12 weeks of gestation in order to reduce the probability of neural tube defects in the fetus.[1,2] If there has been a neural tube defect in a previous pregnancy, 5 mg daily is advised.[2] This is particularly important in the UK, where food is not as yet fortified with folic acid.

References

1. Eichholzer M, Tönz O and Zimmermann R (2006) Folic acid: a public-health challenge. Lancet, 367, 1352–1361. PMID: 16631914
2. Clarke R and Bennett D (2014) Folate and prevention of neural tube defects. BMJ, 349, 7. PMID: 25073785

SBA 16 a Anaemia.

The blood count and film suggest megaloblastic anaemia. It is important to be aware that severe anaemia for any reason can cause retinal haemorrhages. Although there is thrombocytopenia the platelet count is not reduced sufficiently to cause retinal haemorrhages and there is no reason to suspect impaired platelet function. The reference illustrates the retinas of a similar patient with dietary folate deficiency.[1]

Reference

1. Hughes M and Leach M (2006) Dietary folate deficiency and bilateral retinal haemorrhages. *Lancet*, 368, 2155. PMID: 17174707

SBA 17 d Wilson's disease.

The presence of irregularly contracted cells and the positive Heinz body preparation indicate oxidant damage to red cells, Heinz bodies representing oxidised haemoglobin. Glucose-6-phosphate dehydrogenase (G6PD) deficiency would be unlikely because of the ethnic origin and the female gender. Exposure to an exogenous oxidant would be possible but the previous history suggests that there is a chronic disease. The patient was found to have Wilson's disease, the acute haemolysis being due to release of copper from dying liver cells.[1,2] Zieve's syndrome also causes irregularly contracted cells but the patient is teetotal. Autoimmune haemolytic anaemia is excluded by the observation of irregularly contracted cells rather than spherocytes.

References

1. Goldman M and Ali M (1991) Wilson's disease presenting as Heinz-body hemolytic anemia. *CMAJ*, 145, 971–872. PMID: 1913431
2. Bain BJ (1999) Heinz body haemolytic anaemia in Wilson's disease. *Br J Haematol*, 104, 647. PMID: 10192421

SBA 18 e Pure red cell aplasia.

This diagnosis is indicated by the very low reticulocyte count in the face of a severe anaemia. This is among the autoimmune complications of systemic lupus erythematosus (SLE), others including autoimmune haemolytic anaemia and autoimmune thrombocytopenic purpura. Although the creatinine is elevated this would be insufficient to account for such a severe anaemia. Megaloblastic anaemia would be associated with the macrocytosis and would be unlikely to cause severe anaemia with a normal platelet count and white cell count. SLE is more common in people of Afro-Caribbean origin than in Caucasians.[1]

Reference
1. Bartels CM (2014) Systemic lupus erythematosus (SLE). http://emedicine.medscape.com/article/332244-overview (accessed June 2015)

SBA 19 d Henoch–Schönlein purpura.
Palpable purpura is a feature of this condition but not of thrombocytopenic purpura. The distribution of the purpura is also highly suggestive.[1] Henoch–Schönlein purpura is due to a leucocytoclastic vasculitis and often follows an upper respiratory tract infection. Abdominal pain is a common feature whereas haematuria is less common. Arthritis is another common feature.

Reference
1. Saulsbury FT (2007) Clinical update: Henoch-Schönlein purpura. *Lancet*, 369, 976–978. PMID: 17382810

SBA 20 b ESR greater than 40 mm in 1 h.
Three proposed sets of diagnostic criteria for polymyalgia rheumatica all include an ESR greater than 40 mm in 1 h, although 7–20% of patients have been reported to have an ESR below this level.[1] For distinguishing giant cell arteritis from other vasculitides, an ESR greater than 50 mm in 1 h is suggested, with about 11% of patients having a lower level.[1]

Reference
1. Salvarani C, Cantini F and Hunder GG (2008) Polymyalgia rheumatica and giant-cell arteritis. *Lancet*, 372, 234–245. PMID: 18640460

111

SBA 21 e Lupus anticoagulant.

The clinical picture suggests the antiphospholipid syndrome. Livedo reticularis and venous thrombosis are among the more common features of this syndrome. Guidelines for diagnosis include, as laboratory criteria, the presence of anti-β2 glycoprotein 1 antibodies, anti-cardiolipin antibodies or the lupus anticoagulant, in each case the abnormality to be demonstrated on at least two occasions, 12 weeks apart.[1] Of these abnormalities, the lupus anticoagulant is the one that most strongly correlates with thrombosis and with fetal loss.

Reference

1. Ruiz-Irastorza G, Crowther M, Branch W and Khamashta MA (2010) Antiphospholipid syndrome. *Lancet*, 376, 1498–1509. PMID: 20822807

SBA 22 e Vitamin B$_{12}$ deficiency.

The blood film features are those of megaloblastic anaemia. This is more likely to be vitamin B$_{12}$ deficiency than folic acid deficiency, although either would be possible. The clue is in the oval macrocytes and hypersegmented neutrophils. It is important to be aware that schistocytes (red cell fragments) are a feature of severe megaloblastic anaemia and should not lead to a misdiagnosis of a thrombotic microangiopathy.[1,2]

References

1. Bain BJ (2010) Schistocytes in megaloblastic anemia. *Am J Hematol*, 85, 599. PMID: 20201081
2. Routh JK and Koenig SC (2014) Severe vitamin B12 deficiency mimicking thrombotic thrombocytopenic purpura. *Blood*, 124, 1844. PMID: 25346978

SBA 23 b β thalassaemia.

The findings are those of β thalassaemia major.[1] α thalassaemia would either present *in utero* or at birth with hydrops fetalis (deletion of all four alpha genes) or later in life as haemoglobin H disease (deletion of three of four alpha genes), which has a less severe phenotype. Congenital dyserythropoietic anaemia is associated with normocytic or macrocytic red cells and congenital sideroblastic anaemia with a dimorphic blood film. Unless there were a concomitant inflammatory condition, a severe iron deficiency anaemia would be expected to show a serum ferritin of less than 14 µg/l.

Reference

1. Higgs DR, Engel JD and Stamatoyannopoulos G (2012) Thalassaemia. *Lancet*, 379, 373–383. PMID: 21908035

SBA 24 e The haemoglobin A$_{1c}$ is likely to be misleadingly reduced.

There is no reason to doubt the accuracy of the assay but a valid interpretation is not possible because of the shortened red cell life span. This will cause the haemoglobin A$_{1c}$ to be lower than expected at any level of glycaemia. Diabetes mellitus therefore cannot be excluded in this patient.

Haemoglobin A$_{1c}$ can also be misleadingly low in cirrhosis,[1] whereas in iron deficiency anaemia, aplastic anaemia and pure red cell aplasia, it can be misleadingly increased.[2,3] In general, a short red cell life span gives a misleadingly low level and an aged red cell population with a low reticulocyte count gives a misleadingly high level.

In the absence of confounding factors, a haemoglobin A$_{1c}$ <6%/<42 mmol/mol is normal, 6–6.4%/42–47 mmol/mol indicates a high risk of diabetes and levels of 6.5%/48 mmol/mol or more are indicative of diabetes.[3]

References

1. Lahousen T, Hegenbarth K, Ille R, Lipp RW, Krause R, Little RR and Schnedl WJ (2004) Determination of glycated hemoglobin in patients with advanced liver disease. *World J Gastroenterol*, 10, 2284–2286. PMID: 15259084
2. Okawa T, Tsunekawa S, Seino Y, Hamada Y and Oiso Y (2013) Deceptive HbA$_1$c in a patient with pure red cell aplasia. *Lancet*, 382, 366. PMID: 23890045
3. Kilpatrick ES and Atkin SL (2014) Using haemoglobin A1c to diagnose type 2 diabetes or to identify people at high risk of diabetes. *BMJ*, 348, 37–39. PMID: 24769658

SBA 25 e Vitamin K malabsorption.

The condition designated idiopathic bile salt malabsorption may actually be the result of overproduction of bile salts.[1] It leads to diarrhoea and can be ameliorated by administration of colestyramine (previously cholestyramine), an anion-exchange resin that sequesters bile salts. However colestyramine therapy can also lead to malabsorption of fat-soluble vitamins A, D, E and K.[1,2] In this patient vitamin K deficiency has led to the coagulation disorder. The coagulation tests are not compatible with DIC, haemophilia or hyperfibrinolysis. A severe factor X deficiency would provide an explanation but vitamin K deficiency with reductions of factors II, VII, IX and X is more likely given the clinical history.

References

1. Walters J and Pattni SS (2010) Managing bile acid diarrhoea. *Therap Adv Gastroenterol*, 3, 349–357. PMID: 21180614
2. Seguna R, Maw KZ, Lyall HD and Bowles KM (2014) "Haemorrhagic disease of the newborn" 89 years later than expected: vitamin K deficiency bleeding. *Lancet*, 384, 556. PMID: 25110271

SBA 26 a An apparently healthy 70-year-old woman.

Vaccination is advised for healthy elderly people. Although patients with chronic lymphocytic leukaemia are at increased risk of herpes zoster, they may have a sufficient degree of immune insufficiency to preclude administration of this live attenuated vaccine. Similarly, other patients who are immunosuppressed should not be vaccinated.

SBA 27 b Dengue fever.

The combination of clinical and laboratory features is most suggestive of dengue fever. The haematological features of dengue include a normal or low WBC, marked thrombocytopenia and atypical lymphocytes.[1] In dengue haemorrhagic fever there is also a consumptive coagulopathy and the Hb may rise as a result of capillary leakage. In situations where laboratory facilities are limited, a positive tourniquet test can be useful in diagnosis but the same phenomenon can be accidentally demonstrated when the blood pressure is taken. Meningococcal septicaemia can also be complicated by disseminated intravascular coagulation but in that case the neutrophils show striking toxic changes.

Reference

1. Bain BJ and Stubbs MJ (2015) Dengue fever in returning travellers. *Am J Hematol*, 90, 263. PMID: 25839074

SBA 28 d Schistosomiasis.

The clinical features are typical of an allergic response to acute schistosomal infection with entry of parasites through the skin from contaminated water leading to a rash followed by migration of the parasites leading to the other manifestations. This clinical presentation is known as Katayama fever or Katayama syndrome.[1] A travel history is always relevant in a febrile patient, in this instance including enquiry about exposure to lakes and rivers.

Reference
1. Ross AG, Vickers D, Olds GR, Shah SM and McManus DP (2007) Katayama syndrome. *Lancet Infect Dis*, 7, 218–224. PMID: 17317603

SBA 29 d Malaria.

The combination of fever, headache, relative bradycardia for the degree of fever, leucopenia, thrombocytopenia, atypical lymphocytes and elevated lactate dehydrogenase (LDH) suggest malaria. The other infections listed could show some of these features but only malaria would be likely to be associated with an elevated LDH.[1,2]

References
1. Cunha BA (2001) The diagnosis of imported malaria. *Arch Intern Med*, 161, 1926–1928. PMID: 11493157
2. Casalino E, Le Bras J, Chaussin F, Fichelle A and Bouvet E (2002) Predictive factors of malaria in travelers to areas where malaria is endemic. *Arch Intern Med*, 162, 1625–1630. PMID: 12123407

SBA 30 c Anaemia of chronic disease.

Uncomplicated iron deficiency is characterised by a serum ferritin less than 12–15 µg/l. In mixed iron deficiency and anaemia of chronic disease the ferritin is usually between 15 and 50 µg/l. The value in this patient is most suggestive of anaemia of chronic disease.

SBA 31 b Acute myeloid leukaemia.

The high percentage of blast cells in the peripheral blood indicates that this is acute leukaemia (more than 20% is diagnostic of acute leukaemia) and the presence of Auer rods indicates it is acute myeloid leukaemia. The neutrophils show dysplastic features, indicating that they are part of the leukaemic clone.

SBA 32 b Intrinsic factor antibodies.

In view of the blood count and the past history of Hashimoto thyroiditis, the diagnosis you suspect is pernicious anaemia. Serum vitamin B_{12} is much more sensitive and would be measured but the most specific test of those listed is a test for intrinsic factor antibodies, positive in about two-thirds of patients[1]. It should be remembered that with some assays serum vitamin B_{12} can be falsely normal in patients with intrinsic factor antibodies.[2,3] Plasma homocysteine is sensitive but is also elevated in folate deficiency, renal failure, hypothyroidism and vitamin B_6 deficiency.

References

1. Devalia V, Hamilton MS and Molloy AM; British Committee for Standards in Haematology (2014) Guidelines for the diagnosis and treatment of cobalamin and folate disorders. *Br J Haematol*, 166, 496–513. PMID: 24942828
2. Carmel R and Agrawal YP (2012) Failures of cobalamin assays in pernicious anemia. *N Engl J Med*, 367, 385–386. PMID: 22830482
3. Yang DT and Cook RJ (2012) Spurious elevations of vitamin B12 with pernicious anemia. *N Engl J Med*, 366, 1742–1743. PMID: 22551146

SBA 33 c Hypoparathyroidism.

The pattern of calcium deposition is typical of hypoparathyroidism, in this patient resulting from iron deposition in the parathyroid glands. She does have diabetes mellitus resulting from iron deposition in the pancreas but this is not the cause of the cerebral calcification. Appropriate management of iron overload should prevent this complication.

References

1. Mejdoubi M and Zegermann T (2006) Neurological picture. Extensive brain calcification in idiopathic hypoparathyroidism. *J Neurol Neurosurg Psychiatry*, 7, 1328. PMID: 17110747

2. Wong EMM and Dahl M (2013) Basal ganglia calcification in idiopathic hypoparathyroidism. *BCMJ*, 55, 462–465. http://www.bcmj.org/articles/basal-ganglia-calcification-idiopathic-hypoparathyroidism (accessed June 2015)

SBA 34 e Primary myelofibrosis.

The blood count and blood film would be compatible with either primary myelofibrosis or metastatic cancer involving the bone marrow. The significant splenomegaly points to the former diagnosis. Although the platelet count is increased, essential thrombocythaemia would not be expected to show either a leucoerythroblastic blood film or marked splenomegaly.

SBA 35 d Sickle cell-related intrahepatic cholestasis.

This condition results from sickling within hepatic sinusoids leading to vascular stasis and hypoxic injury to hepatocytes with resultant swelling leading in turn to intracanalicular cholestasis.[1] The condition may progress over time to liver failure.

Reference

1. Gardner K, Suddle A, Kane P, O'Grady J, Heaton N, Bomford A and Thein SL (2014) How we treat sickle hepatopathy and liver transplantation in adults. *Blood*, 123, 2302–2307. PMID: 24565828

SBA 36 a Atypical haemolytic uraemic syndrome (aHUS).

The patient has a microangiopathic haemolytic anaemia with thrombocytopenia. The history of diarrhoea is not enough to assign a diagnosis of HUS at an atypical age and in the absence of Shiga toxin. The ADAMTS13 assay excludes a diagnosis of TTP. A diagnosis of aHUS is most likely and investigation for complement mutations is indicated.[1,2]

References

1. Feng S, Eyler SJ, Zhang Y, Maga T, Nester CM, Kroll MH *et al.* (2013) Partial ADAMTS13 deficiency in atypical hemolytic uremic syndrome. *Blood*, 122, 1487–1493. PMID: 23847193
2. Cataland SR and Wu HM (2014) How I treat: the clinical differentiation and initial treatment of adult patients with atypical hemolytic uremic syndrome. *Blood*, 123, 2478–2484. PMID: 24599547

SBA 37 d Rasburicase.

The clinical and laboratory features indicate tumour lysis syndrome with early signs of acute renal injury. Urinary alkalinisation is not indicated since xanthine, hypoxanthine and calcium precipitate in the kidneys in alkaline conditions. Allopurinol may be used in prophylaxis but is not recommended in overt tumour lysis syndrome. Calcium gluconate should be administered since the hypocalcaemia is symptomatic, but with the aim of alleviating the symptoms rather than normalising the calcium level. Haemofiltration or haemodialysis is preferred to peritoneal dialysis since it is more rapidly efficacious but in this patient there is not yet an indication for this. Since the patient is Northern European you do not need to be concerned about the possibility that he is deficient in glucose-6-phosphate dehydrogenase and might suffer haemolysis after rasburicase and this is therefore indicated.[1,2]

References

1. Cairo MS, Coiffier B, Reiter A and Younes A; TLS Expert Panel (2010) Recommendations for the evaluation of risk and prophylaxis of tumour lysis syndrome (TLS) in adults and children with malignant diseases: an expert TLS panel consensus. *Br J Haematol*, 149, 578–586. PMID: 20331465
2. Jones GL, Will A, Jackson GH, Webb N and Rule S; British Committee for Standards in Haematology (2015) Guidelines for the management of tumour lysis syndrome in adults and children with haematological malignancies. *Br J Haematol*, 93, 1877–1885. PMID: 18838473

SBA 38 a Measure D dimer.

The Wells' score is a method of determining the clinical probability of a DVT.[1] If the Wells' score is 0 or 1 DVT is, in general, unlikely; D dimer should be measured and if it is normal no further investigation or intervention is indicated. However if there is a history of previous thromboembolism one point should be added to the score.[2,3] This patient then scores 1 so again no further investigation or treatment is indicated. The Wells' score has been recently found to be invalid in patients with cancer.[2]

References

1. Wells PS, Anderson DR, Rodger M, Forgie M, Kearon C, Dreyer J *et al.* (2003) Evaluation of D-dimer in the diagnosis of deep-vein thrombosis. *N Engl J Med*, 349, 1227–1235. PMID: 14507948

2. Geersing GJ, Zuithoff NP, Kearon C, Anderson DR, Ten Cate-Hoek AJ, Elf JL *et al*. (2014) Exclusion of deep vein thrombosis using the Wells rule in clinically important subgroups: individual patient data meta-analysis. *BMJ*. 348, 12. PMID: 24615063
3. Iorio A and Douketis JD (2014) Ruling out DVT using the Wells rule and a D-dimer test. *BMJ*, 348, 8. PMID: 24615174

SBA 39 c Cholesterol embolisation.

The clinical features, the eosinophilia and the timing of the deterioration suggest cholesterol embolisation. This can be provoked by anticoagulation as a result of interference with the protective clot over ulcerated atheromatous plaques of the aorta. This syndrome rarely follows initiation of warfarin, occurring 3–8 weeks later, but thrombolytic therapy can also be implicated. This case was reported and discussed by Mooney and Joseph.[1] Diagnosis can be confirmed by the observation of clefts representing dissolved cholesterol crystals in renal, bone marrow or other biopsy specimens with a surrounding foreign body reaction.[2]

References
1. Mooney T and Joseph P (2014) Purple toes syndrome following stroke thrombolysis and warfarin therapy. *Intern Med J*, 44, 107–108. PMID: 24450530
2. Dupont PJ, Lightstone L, Clutterbuck EJ, Gaskin G, Pusey CD, Cook T and Warrens AN (2000) Cholesterol emboli syndrome. *Br Med J*, 321, 1065–1067. PMID: 11053182

SBA 40 b Fluid restriction.

The patient has hyponatraemia and low serum osmolality with an inappropriately high urine osmolality (should be less than 100 in the face of serum hypo-osmolality). This indicates the syndrome of inappropriate secretion of antidiuretic hormone (SIADH).[1] This results from a failure of suppression of ADH secretion in response to fluid intake and a low serum osmolality so that fluid is retained, urine osmolality is inappropriately high and serum osmolality falls further. Among the many known causes is administration of vincristine or cyclophosphamide. Hypertonic saline infusion is only used for patients with severe acute symptoms. Treatment in this patient who does not have severe symptoms can be by fluid restriction (e.g. to 500 or 1,000 ml/day). Correction of hyponatraemia should be slow as rapid correction can lead to central pontine myelinolysis. Tolvaptan is an orally active vasopressin V_2-receptor antagonist which promotes excretion of solute-free water. Introduction of this drug could be considered if the serum sodium does not rise by 2 mmol/l in the first 24 hours of fluid restriction.[2]

References

1. Thomas CP, Syndrome of inappropriate antidiuretic hormone secretion. http://emedicine. medscape.com/article/246650-overview (accessed June 2015)
2. Schrier RW, Gross P, Gheorghiade M, Berl T, Verbalis JG, Czerwiec FS and Orlandi C; SALT Investigators (2006) Tolvaptan, a selective oral vasopressin V2-receptor antagonist, for hyponatremia. *N Engl J Med*, 355, 2099–2112. PMID: 17105757

SBA 41 b Intravenous fluids 3 l/m^2/d plus allopurinol.

A patient at high risk of tumour lysis syndrome would normally receive rasburicase but this is contraindicated in this patient because of his G6PD deficiency. He should therefore receive allopurinol. Urinary alkalinisation is not recommended since although it increases the solubility of uric acid it decreases solubility of calcium phosphate and may cause xanthine precipitation.[1] Potassium should not be added to the intravenous fluids.

Reference

1. Howard SC, Jones DP and Pui CH (2011) The tumor lysis syndrome. *N Engl J Med*, 364, 1844–1854. PMID: 21561350

SBA 42 e Temporal artery biopsy followed by prednisolone in a dose of 40–60 mg daily.

Although the clinical features are strongly suggestive of temporal arteritis, urgent confirmation of the diagnosis is necessary. Once the biopsy is done, it would be reasonable to commence treatment while awaiting histological confirmation. The biopsy specimen should measure 1.5–3 cm but there is little benefit in bilateral biopsies and this is not recommended.[1] Oral prednisolone is the preferred treatment.[1] The features are not those of migraine and ibuprofen or diclofenac would not be appropriate.

Reference

1. Salvarani C, Cantini F and Hunder GG (2008) Polymyalgia rheumatica and giant-cell arteritis. *Lancet*, 372, 234–245. PMID: 18640460

SBA 43 d Molecular analysis for *JAK2* mutation.
The red cell indices would be consistent with either thalassaemia trait or iron deficient polycythaemia except that the MCHC is reduced, a feature of iron deficiency but not of thalassaemia trait. β thalassaemia is also unlikely in a Northern European Caucasian. In addition, the elevated platelet count and WBC point to the possibility of a myeloproliferative neoplasm, most likely iron-deficient polycythaemia vera. This is very likely to be confirmed by molecular analysis for the *JAK2* V617F mutation, detected in 95% of patients with polycythaemia vera. A bone marrow aspirate alone could confirm the iron deficiency but for further elucidation of the diagnosis would always be combined with a trephine biopsy. A therapeutic trial of iron would be very unwise since a rise in the Hb could lead to further vascular events.

SBA 44 b Computed tomography pulmonary angiogram.
The patient's history and investigations suggest an antiphospholipid syndrome, which can cause both arterial and venous thrombosis. However the urgent requirement is to confirm that her recent symptoms are due to a pulmonary embolus rather than pneumonia and to commence anticoagulant therapy. A computed tomography pulmonary angiogram is the preferred investigation for this purpose.

SBA 45 c Serum tryptase.
Recurrent anaphylaxis, often unprovoked, should raise the suspicion of systemic mastocytosis.[1,2] The most relevant management step listed is a serum tryptase estimation.[3] A concentration persistently above 20 ng/ml is an important diagnostic criterion, assay not being performed immediately after an attack. The patient also requires a bone marrow aspirate and trephine biopsy. It is possible that his history of indigestion is due to peptic ulcer disease resulting from histamine excess. Patients with systemic mastocytosis often have eosinophilia and sometimes monocytosis.

References
1. Müller UR and Haeberli G (2009) The problem of anaphylaxis and mastocytosis. *Curr Allergy Asthma Rep*, 9, 64–70. PMID: 19063827

2. Gülen T, Hägglund H, Dahlén SE, Sander B, Dahlén B and Nilsson G (2014) Flushing, fatigue, and recurrent anaphylaxis: a delayed diagnosis of mastocytosis. *Lancet*, 383, 1608. PMID: 24792857

3. Horny H-P, Metcalfe DD, Bennett JM, Bain BJ, Akin C, Escribano L and Valent P. Mastocytosis. *In* Swerdlow SH, Campo E, Harris NL, Jaffe ES, Pileri SA, Stein H, Thiele J and Vardiman JW (Eds) *World Health Organization Classification of Tumours of Haematopoietic and Lymphoid Tissues*, 4th Edn, IARC Press, Lyon, 2008, pp 54–63.

SBA 46 e Warfarin or non-vitamin K antagonist oral anticoagulant.

Current NICE guidelines advise that anticoagulation should be offered to patients with a $CHAD_2DS_2$-VASc score of 2 or more, taking the risk of bleeding into account.[1,2] Either warfarin or a non-vitamin K antagonist oral anticoagulant would be appropriate. Aspirin is not recommended for stroke prevention in this setting.

References

1. Jones C, Pollit V, Fitzmaurice D and Cowan C; Guideline Development Group (2014). The management of atrial fibrillation: summary of updated NICE guidance. *BMJ*, 348, 34–37. PMID: 24948694

2. National Institute for Health and Care Excellence (2014) Atrial fibrillation: managing atrial fibrillation. http://www.nice.org.uk/guidance/CG180 (accessed June 2015)

SBA 47 d Rivaroxaban is relevant and she is likely to be fully anticoagulated.

Rivaroxaban is a direct acting factor Xa inhibitor, which she is taking because of her atrial fibrillation. The effect of this drug on coagulation tests is reagent-dependent. There tends to be more effect on the pro-thrombin time (PT) than on the activated partial thromboplastin time (APTT).[1] Normal or near normal test results do not indicate a lack of an anticoagulant effect and as the patient is reported to have taken her medications it is likely that she is fully anticoagulated. It is important to be aware of the new, direct acting oral anticoagulants, both because of their relevance to invasive procedures and because agents for reversal are under development, for use in the case of haemorrhage. In the case of rivaroxaban the reversal agent is andexanet, a recombinant molecule that resembles factor Xa and mops up the factor Xa inhibitor.

Reference

1. Kitchen S, Gray E, Mackie I, Baglin T and Makris M; BCSH committee (2014) Measurement of non-coumarin anticoagulants and their effects on tests of Haemostasis: Guidance from the British Committee for Standards in Haematology. *Br J Haematol*, 166, 830–841. PMID: 24930477

SBA 48 b Four-factor prothrombin complex plus vitamin K.

Prothrombin complex containing factors II, VII, IX and X, in combination with vitamin K is recommended.[1,2]

References

1. Keeling D, Baglin T, Tait C, Watson H, Perry D, Baglin C et al.; British Committee for Standards in Haematology(2011) Guidelines on oral anticoagulation with warfarin - fourth edition. *Br J Haematol*, 154, 311–324. PMID: 21671894
2. Rodgers GM (2012) Prothrombin complex concentrates in emergency bleeding disorders. *Am J Hematol*, 87, 898–902. PMID: 22648513

SBA 49 d Factor XI deficiency

Only factor XI deficiency and factor XII deficiency cause prolongation of the APTT without prolongation of the PT. However factor XII deficiency does not cause haemorrhage. Deficiency of factor VIII or IX would actually be more likely since they are more common but they are not among the options offered.

SBA 50 b No specific treatment

Patients with liver disease have not only reduction of the concentration of many coagulation factors but also a reduction in the concentration of naturally occurring anticoagulants.[1] The International Normalised Ratio (INR) therefore does not have the same significance as in a patient receiving vitamin K antagonists. This patient requires no specific management of his coagulation status prior to surgery.

Reference

1. Roberts JR and Bambha K (2014) Balanced coagulopathy in cirrhosis-clinical implications: a teachable moment. *JAMA Intern Med*, 174, 1723–1724. PMID: 25201536

SBA 51 d Sézary syndrome.

The generalised erythroderma and the CD25 negativity do not favour adult T-cell leukaemia/lymphoma (ATLL). The clinical features and the CD7 negativity do not favour T-prolymphocytic leukaemia (T-PLL). The skin lesions are not typical of mycosis fungoides, in which erythroderma is quite uncommon; circulating lymphoma cells are also uncommon in mycosis fungoides. The cutaneous manifestations, alopecia, generalised lymphadenopathy (likely to be dermatopathic lymphadenopathy) and immunophenotype are compatible with Sézary syndrome, although CD2 is often positive. It would be inappropriate to suggest a diagnosis of idiopathic hypereosinophilic syndrome in a patient with a manifest T-cell neoplasm.

The reference given discusses the immunophenotype and diagnostic criteria for Sézary syndrome.[1]

Reference

1. Carter JB, Barnes JA, Niell BL and Nardi V (2013) Case records of the Massachusetts General Hospital. Case 24-2013. A 53-year-old woman with erythroderma, pruritus, and lymphadenopathy. *N Engl J Med*, 369, 559–569. PMID: 23924007

SBA 52 b Imatinib 200–300 mg daily.

The features described are typical of chronic myelogeneous leukaemia in chronic phase. Hyperviscosity is unusual with a WBC less than $200 \times 10^9/l$ and there were no relevant features on history or physical examination so leukapheresis is not indicated. Imatinib is the first line treatment indicated and in a child the appropriate dose would be 200–300 mg daily.[1]

Reference

1. de la Fuente J, Baruchel A, Biondi A, de Bont E, Dresse MF, Suttorp M, Millot F; International BFM Group (iBFM) Study Group Chronic Myeloid Leukaemia Committee (2014) Managing children with chronic myeloid leukaemia (CML): recommendations for the management of CML in children and young people up to the age of 18 years. *Br J Haematol*, 167, 33–47. PMID: 24976289

SBA 53 b Combination chemotherapy followed by involved field radiotherapy.

Meta-analysis and systematic review have shown that combination chemotherapy followed by involved field radiotherapy shows improved tumour control and overall survival when compared with chemotherapy alone.[1] The patient did not actually need a trephine biopsy as only about 1% of patients with limited stage disease after positron emission tomography/computed tomography (PET/CT) scanning are found to have bone marrow disease.[2]

References

1. Herbst C, Rehan FA, Brillant C, Bohlius J, Skoetz N, Schulz H *et al.* (2010) Combined modality treatment improves tumor control and overall survival in patients with early stage Hodgkin's lymphoma: a systematic review. *Haematologica*, 95, 494–500. PMID: 19951972
2. Townsend W and Linch D (2012) Hodgkin's lymphoma in adults. *Lancet*, 380, 836–847. PMID: 22835602

SBA 54 e Molecular analysis for a *JAK2* exon 12 mutation.

The features described are most suggestive of polycythaemia vera and since *JAK2* V617F has not been detected, a *JAK2* exon 12 mutation is suspected.[1] An inherited cause of polycythaemia is less likely. The reduced serum erythropoietin makes respiratory and renal causes of polycythaemia unlikely. *CALR* mutation is a feature of essential thrombocythaemia and primary myelofibrosis rather than polycythaemia vera. There is one report indicating that polycythaemia vera with a *JAK2* exon 12 mutation is much more common in Chinese than in Caucasian patients.[2]

References

1. Lakey MA, Pardanani A, Hoyer JD, Nguyen PL, Lasho TL, Tefferi A, Hanson CA (2010) Bone marrow morphologic features in polycythemia vera with JAK2 exon 12 mutations. *Am J Clin Pathol*, 133, 942–948. PMID: 20472853
2. Yeh YM, Chen YL, Cheng HY, Su WC, Chow NH, Chen TY and Ho CL (2010) High percentage of *JAK2* exon 12 mutation in Asian patients with polycythemia vera. *Am J Clin Pathol*, 134, 266–170. PMID: 20660330

SBA 55 a Acquired von Willebrand disease.

This is acquired von Willebrand disease resulting from Wilms tumour. This is the malignancy most often associated with acquired von Willebrand disease and acquired von Willebrand disease is found in about 8% of newly diagnosed patients with Wilms tumour.[1] The mechanism is adsorption of von Willebrand factor (VWF) by the tumour.

This question could well be considered too esoteric for the FRCPath examination but the wrong answers can be excluded by studying the test results carefully[2].

References

1. Callaghan MU, Wong TE and Federici AB (2013) Treatment of acquired von Willebrand syndrome in childhood. *Blood*, 122, 2019–2022. PMID: 23878141
2. Laffan MA, Lester W, O'Donnell JS, Will A, Tait RC, Goodeve A *et al.* (2014) The diagnosis and management of von Willebrand disease: a United Kingdom Haemophilia Centre Doctors Organization guideline approved by the British Committee for Standards in Haematology. *Br J Haematol*, 167, 453–465. PMID: 25113304

SBA 56 e The eculizumab therapy is unmasking C3 binding to red cells.

Eculizumab is an anti-C5 monoclonal antibody, which blocks the action of C5.[1,2] Its use may unmask binding of C3 to red cells. Because the action of C5 is blocked, these cells are no longer lysed intravascularly. However, the direct antiglobulin test may become positive and chronic extravascular haemolysis can occur.

References

1. Hill A, Rother RP, Arnold L, Kelly R, Cullen MJ, Richards SJ and Hillmen P (2010) Eculizumab prevents intravascular hemolysis in patients with paroxysmal nocturnal hemoglobinuria and unmasks low-level extravascular hemolysis occurring through C3 opsonization. *Haematologica*, 95, 567–573. PMID: 20145265
2. Luzzatto L, Risitano AM and Notaro R (2010) Paroxysmal nocturnal hemoglobinuria and eculizumab. *Haematologica*, 95, 523–526. PMID: 20378572

SBA 57 d Transfusion of blood intended for another patient.

Patients should give valid consent for transfusion and this requires explaining the risks and benefits and providing written information to inform their decision.

The NHSBT (NHS Blood and Transplant) information leaflet 'Will I need a blood transfusion?' is a very helpful way of standardising information and it states, 'One of the most important ways of achieving a safe transfusion is to make sure you get the right blood. You can help reduce the small risk of being given the wrong blood by asking your nurse or doctor to check that it is the right blood for you.'

This information leaflet also gives the current estimated risk of viral transmission and states 'Hepatitis B might be passed on by fewer than 1 in 1.3 million blood donations and the risk is many times smaller for HIV (1 in 6.5 million) and hepatitis C (1 in 28 million) (figures published October 2012).'[1,2]

References

1. SaBTO Patient Consent for Blood Transfusion October 2011. Published on the UK government website https://www.gov.uk/government/publications/patient-consent-for-blood-transfusion (accessed June 2015)
2. NHSBT information leaflets can be found on the NHSBT Hospital and Science website. http://hospital.blood.co.uk (Similar leaflets are provided by the Welsh, Scottish and Northern Ireland blood services.)

SBA 58 a Arrange molecular analysis for a *CALR* mutation and *BCR-ABL1*.

The differential diagnosis is between essential thrombocythaemia, chronic myelogenous leukaemia and prefibrotic myelofibrosis. Because of the therapeutic implications, it is important to confirm or exclude chronic myelogenous leukaemia by an analysis for *BCR-ABL1*. A diagnosis of essential thrombocythaemia cannot be made until *BCR-ABL1* has been excluded. However it is more probable that the patient described has essential thrombocythaemia with a *CALR* mutation (found in a quarter of patients with essential thrombocythaemia) and therefore simultaneous analysis for *CALR* mutation and *BCR-ABL1* would be a sensible approach.[1-3] *JAK2* exon 12 mutation is only relevant if polycythaemia vera is suspected. The normal Hb and MCV are against a diagnosis of the 5q– syndrome. An *MPL* mutation is found in only a minority of patients (about 5%) with essential thrombocythaemia so is less likely to be useful.

127

References

1. Harrison CN, Bareford D, Butt N, Campbell P, Conneally E, Drummond M *et al.*; British Committee for Standards in Haematology (2010) Guideline for investigation and management of adults and children presenting with a thrombocytosis. *Br J Haematol*, 149, 352–375. PMID: 20331456
2. Harrison CN, Butt N, Campbell P, Conneally E, Drummond M, Green AR *et al.* (2013) Diagnostic pathway for the investigation of thrombocytosis. *Br J Haematol*, 161, 604–606. PMID: 23480550
3. Cazzola M and Kralovics R (2014) From Janus kinase 2 to calreticulin: the clinically relevant genomic landscape of myeloproliferative neoplasms. *Blood*, 123, 3714–3719. PMID: 24786775

SBA 59 d Top-up transfusion to achieve an Hb of 100 g/l.

The TAPS randomised controlled trial found preoperative transfusion aiming for an Hb of 100 g/l to be beneficial, in comparison with no transfusion, in patients with sickle cell anaemia having medium risk surgery (and possibly in those having low risk surgery).[1] In this trial, patients with an Hb less than 90 g/l had a top-up transfusion and those with an Hb above this level had a partial exchange transfusion. A reduction in serious adverse events and clinically important complications, particularly acute chest syndrome, was demonstrated in the whole group, of whom 81% were having medium rather than low risk surgery. An earlier randomised controlled trial had found exchange transfusion aiming for a haemoglobin S of less than 30% to have no advantage over top-up transfusion aiming for an Hb of 100 g/l.[2]

References

1. Howard J, Malfroy M, Llewelyn C, Choo L, Hodge R, Johnson T *et al.* (2013) The Transfusion Alternatives Preoperatively in Sickle Cell Disease (TAPS) study: a randomised, controlled, multicentre clinical trial. *Lancet*, 381, 930–938. PMID: 23352054
2. Vichinsky EP, Haberkern CM, Neumayr L, Earles AN, Black D, Koshy M *et al.* (1995) A comparison of conservative and aggressive transfusion regimens in the perioperative management of sickle cell disease. The Preoperative Transfusion in Sickle Cell Disease Study Group. *N Engl J Med*, 333, 206–213. PMID: 7791837

SBA 60 d Ruxolitinib.

Ruxolitinib is indicated in patients with primary myelofibrosis who have symptomatic splenomegaly or other disease-related symptoms that are reducing quality of life.[1–3] There is amelioration of symptoms and the

COMFORT-II trial also showed improved survival.[2] Ruxolitinib is useful whether or not a *JAK2* V617F mutation is present.[1]

References

1. Reilly JT, McMullin MF, Beer PA, Butt N, Conneally E, Duncombe AS *et al.* (2014) Use of JAK inhibitors in the management of myelofibrosis: a revision of the British Committee for Standards in Haematology Guidelines for Investigation and Management of Myelofibrosis 2012. *Br J Haematol*, 167, 418–420. PMID: 24961987
2. Cervantes F, Vannucchi AM, Kiladjian JJ, Al-Ali HK, Sirulnik A, Stalbovskaya V *et al.* (2013) Three-year efficacy, safety, and survival findings from COMFORT-II, a phase 3 study comparing ruxolitinib with best available therapy for myelofibrosis. *Blood*, 122, 4047–4053. PMID: 24174625
3. Passamonti F, Maffioli M, Cervantes F, Vannucchi AM, Morra E, Barbui T *et al.* (2014) Impact of ruxolitinib on the natural history of primary myelofibrosis: a comparison of the DIPSS and the COMFORT-2 cohorts. *Blood*, 123, 1833–1835. PMID: 24443442

SBA 61 c Juvenile myelomonocytic leukaemia.

The features are all those of juvenile myelomonocytic leukaemia. Erythropoiesis may show reversion to fetal characteristics including a high percentage of haemoglobin F, increased expression of i antigen, reduced carbonic anhydrase and reduced or even absent haemoglobin A_2.[1] The pulmonary features are the result of peribronchial and interstitial infiltration.[2]

References

1. Bain BJ. *Leukaemia Diagnosis*, 4th Edn, Wiley-Blackwell, Oxford, 2010.
2. Niemeyer CM (2014) RAS diseases in children. *Haematologica*, 99, 1653–1662. PMID: 25420281

SBA 62 d Horse antithymocyte globulin plus ciclosporin.

The diagnosis is aplastic anaemia. Moderate dysplasia is not unexpected and does not suggest a diagnosis of myelodysplastic syndrome. Horse antithymocyte globulin is more effective than rabbit anti-thymocyte globulin so, if available, is preferred and should be combined with ciclosporin since the combination is more effective than antithymocyte globulin alone; rabbit antithymocyte globulin or alemtuzumab may be useful as second line treatment in patients who fail to respond.[1,2]

References

1. Gafter-Gvili A, Ram R, Gurion R, Paul M, Yeshurun M, Raanani P and Shpilberg O (2008) ATG plus cyclosporine reduces all–cause mortality in patients with severe aplastic anemia – systematic review and meta-analysis. *Acta Haematol*, 120, 237–243. PMID: 19246887
2. Young NS (2013) Current concepts in pathogenesis and treatment of aplastic anemia. *Hematology Am Soc Hematol Educ Program*, 2013, 76–81. PMID: 24319166 http://asheducation-book.hematologylibrary.org/content/2013/1/76.long (accessed June 2015)

SBA 63 a Autoimmune lymphoproliferative syndrome.

The combination of multiple autoimmune manifestations and the presence of CD4-CD8- ('double negative') lymphocytes is indicative of the autoimmune lymphoproliferative syndrome (ALPS).[1,2] The presence of more than 5% of double negative lymphocytes has been suggested as a criterion for this diagnosis. Evans syndrome would not be a wrong diagnosis but would not explain the neutropenia and the abnormal lymphocyte population. SLE similarly would not explain the abnormal lymphocyte population.

References

1. Teachey DT, Seif AE and Grupp SA (2010) Advances in the management and understanding of autoimmune lymphoproliferative syndrome (ALPS). *Br J Haematol*, 148, 205–216. PMID: 19930184
2. Iyengar SR, Ebb DH, Yuan Q, Shailam R and Bhan AK (2013) Case records of the Massachusetts General Hospital. Case 27-2013. A 6.5-month-old boy with fever, rash, and cytopenias. *N Engl J Med*, 369, 853–863. PMID: 23984733

SBA 64 a Blastic plasmacytoid dendritic cell neoplasm

The immunophenotype is that of blastic plasmacytoid dendritic cell neoplasm.[1] The clinical history is compatible with this diagnosis, since presentation is often with skin involvement.

Reference

1. Cronin DM, George TI, Reichard KK and Sundram UN (2012) Immunophenotypic analysis of myeloperoxidase-negative leukemia cutis and blastic plasmacytoid dendritic cell neoplasm. *Am J Clin Pathol*, 137, 367–376. PMID: 22338048

SBA 65 a Adult T-cell leukaemia/lymphoma.

The clinical features are strongly suggestive of ATLL. Surface membrane CD3 is often not expressed but these are nevertheless mature T cells. CD25 expression and lack of expression of CD7 are expected.[1-3]

References

1. Matutes E, Bain BJ and Wotherspoon A. *An Atlas of Investigation and Diagnosis: Lymphoid Malignancies*. Clinical Publishing, Oxford, 2007.
2. Parker A, Bain B, Devereux S, Gatter K, Jack A, Matutes E *et al*. British Committee for Standards in Haematology (2010) Best practice in lymphoma diagnosis and reporting. http://www.bcshguidelines.com/documents/lymphoma_diagnosis_bcsh_042010.pdf (accessed June 2015)
3. Parker A, Bain B, Devereux S, Gatter K, Jack A, Matutes E *et al*. British Committee for Standards in Haematology (2010) Best practice in lymphoma diagnosis and reporting: specific disease appendix. http://www.bcshguidelines.com/documents/lymphoma_disease_app_bcsh_042010.pdf (accessed June 2015)

SBA 66 e Von Willebrand factor-containing plasma-derived concentrate.

The findings are those of Von Willebrand disease, type III, which is characterised by a severe quantitative deficiency of von Willebrand factor. With such severe disease, desmopressin would be ineffective and tranexamic acid alone would offer little benefit. Recombinant factor VIII alone is not recommended since the von Willebrand molecule is needed to prolong the half-life of factor VIII. A concentrate containing von Willebrand factor is needed.[1,2] Depending on the individual concentrate chosen, supplementation with factor VIII may be necessary if there is serious acute bleeding as it may otherwise be more than 12 hours before factor VIII rises to normal levels.[2]

References

1. Federici AB and James P (2012) Current management of patients with severe von Willebrand disease type 3: a 2012 update. *Acta Haematol*, 128, 88–99. PMID: 22722677
2. Laffan MA, Lester W, O'Donnell JS, Will A, Tait RC, Goodeve A *et al*. (2014) The diagnosis and management of von Willebrand disease: a United Kingdom Haemophilia Centre Doctors Organization guideline approved by the British Committee for Standards in Haematology. *Br J Haematol*, 167, 453–465. PMID: 25113304

SBA 67 a B-cell lymphoma, unclassifiable, with features intermediate between diffuse large B-cell lymphoma and Burkitt lymphoma.

Although this a 'double hit' lymphoma,[1] this is not a WHO diagnosis. Burkitt lymphoma cells express CD10 and BCL6 (germinal centre phenotype) but not BCL2, and the proliferation fraction approaches 100% so the diagnosis is not Burkitt lymphoma.[2]

References
1. Barnes JA, Abramson JS, Scott JA and Sohani AR (2013) Case 35-2013: a 77-year-old man with confusion and malaise. *N Engl J Med*, 369, 1946–1957. PMID: 24224628
2. Kluin PM, Harris NL, Stein H. Leoncini L, Raphaël M, Campo E and Jaffe ES, B-cell lymphoma, unclassifiable, with features intermediate between diffuse large B-cell lymphoma and Burkitt lymphoma. *In* Swerdlow SH, Campo E, Harris NL, Jaffe ES, Pileri SA, Stein H, Thiele J and Vardiman J (Eds) *WHO Classification of Tumours of Haematopoietic and Lymphoid Tissues*. IARC, Lyon, 2008, pp 265–266.

SBA 68 d Rituximab.

Corticosteroid and alkylating agents have a low rate of response in cold haemagglutinin disease. Splenectomy is not generally useful. Rituximab has a response rate of 50–80% with about half of patients not needing further treatment.[1,2]

References
1. Berentsen S (2011) How I manage cold agglutinin disease. *Br J Haematol*, 153, 309–317. PMID: 21385173
2. Swiecicki PL, Hegerova LT and Gertz MA (2013) Cold agglutinin disease. *Blood*, 122, 1114–1121. PMID: 23757733

SBA 69 c Doxycycline.

Many cases of ocular adnexal MALT-type lymphoma appear to be aetiologically related to *Chlamydophila psittaci* (previously *Chlamydia psittaci*). There is a significant response rate to antibiotic therapy, mainly doxycycline. In a total of 213 patients treated in seven trials the complete response rate was 18% and the partial response rate 27%.[1] Response is more likely when *Chlamydophila psittaci* is identified but is not confined to these patients so prior culture does not appear necessary.

Reference

1. Kiesewetter B and Raderer M (2013) Antibiotic therapy in nongastrointestinal MALT lymphoma: a review of the literature. *Blood*, 122, 1350–1357. PMID: 23770778

SBA 70 a Clusters of CD34-positive cells in biopsy sections

Macrocytosis and a low absolute reticulocyte count may be seen in both hypoplastic myelodysplastic syndrome (MDS) and aplastic anaemia. The presence of a minor PNH clone is more consistent with aplastic anaemia than MDS. The cytogenetic findings given are not sufficient to define a clonal cytogenetic abnormality so are unhelpful and, in addition, abnormal clones can appear and disappear in aplastic anaemia. The presence of clusters of CD34-positive cells indicates increased blast cells and favours hypoplastic MDS.[1]

Reference

1. Orazi A, Albitar M, Heerema NA, Haskins S and Neiman RS (1997) Hypoplastic myelodysplastic syndromes can be distinguished from acquired aplastic anemia by CD34 and PRNA immunostaining of bone marrow biopsy specimens. *Am J Clin Pathol*, 107, 268–274.

SBA 71 e Therapy-related myeloid neoplasm.

In view of the previous history, the diagnosis is therapy-related myeloid neoplasm rather than refractory anaemia with excess of blasts 2. The WHO classification groups together therapy-related acute myeloid leukaemia and therapy-related MDS since the prognosis of the latter is as adverse as that of the former. The cytogenetic abnormality is one known to be associated with prior exposure to topoisomerase II-interactive drugs.[1]

Reference

1. Gabriel IH, Abdalla SH, Ryley S and Bain BJ (2007) Teaching case 34: acute leukaemia in a patient with a previous history of breast cancer. *Leuk Lymphoma*, 48, 403–405. PMID: 17325903

SBA 72 e Recombinant factor VIIa OR activated prothrombin complex, followed by cyclophosphamide and corticosteroids.

Recombinant factor VIIa and activated prothrombin complex are equally efficacious and one or other is the preferred initial treatment.[1,2] High dose human factor VIII is less efficacious. Porcine factor VIII is no longer available. Desmopressin is only of use in patients with a low titre inhibitor. Initial treatment should be followed by immunosuppression. Corticosteroids plus cyclophosphamide are more efficacious than corticosteroids alone.

References
1. Baudo F, Collins P, Huth-Kühne A, Lévesque H, Marco P, Nemes L *et al.*; EACH2 registry contributors (2012) Management of bleeding in acquired hemophilia A: results from the European Acquired Haemophilia (EACH2) Registry. *Blood*, 120, 39–46. PMID: 22618709
2. Collins PW (2012) Therapeutic challenges in acquired factor VIII deficiency. http://asheducationbook.hematologylibrary.org/content/2012/1/369.long (accessed June 2015)

SBA 73 c Plasma exchange followed by eculizumab.

The differential diagnosis includes TTP as well as aHUS and patients should be started on plasma exchange while awaiting ADAMTS13 results. Patients with TTP usually have a platelet count of less than 30×10^9/l and a serum creatinine of less than 220 µmol/l, which can predict an ADAMTS13 of less than 10%.[1-4] Except when the underlying mutation is in *MCP*, patients with aHUS have a high rate of end stage renal disease unless they receive eculizumab. Immunosuppressive therapy would be indicated only in patients in whom aHUS is due to autoantibodies to complement factor H. Meningococcal vaccination is required in any patient who is to be given eculizumab.

References
1. Noris M and Remuzzi G (2009) Atypical hemolytic-uremic syndrome. *N Engl J Med*, 361, 1676–1687. PMID: 19846853
2. Bentley MJ, Lehman CM, Blaylock RC, Wilson AR and Rodgers GM (2010) The utility of patient characteristics in predicting severe ADAMTS13 deficiency and response to plasma exchange. *Transfusion*, 50, 1654–1664. PMID: 20412532

3. Nester CM and Thomas CP (2013) Atypical hemolytic uremic syndrome: what is it, how is it diagnosed, and how is it treated? http://asheducationbook.hematologylibrary.org/content/2012/1/617.long (accessed June 2015)

4. Cataland SR and Wu HM (2014) How I treat: the clinical differentiation and initial treatment of adult patients with atypical hemolytic uremic syndrome. *Blood*, 123, 2478–2484. PMID: 24599547

SBA 74 e Withholding the second dose of desmopressin and no encouragement of fluid intake.

In this reported patient, the second dose of desmopressin was administered, the sodium fell to 117 mmol/l and the patient suffered hyponatraemic seizures.[1] Low urine output is expected after desmopressin administration and does not indicate volume depletion. Fluid intake should not have been increased and the need for the second dose of desmopressin should have been reviewed. Current UK guidelines advise restricting fluid intake to 1 l per day when desmopressin is administered.[2]

References

1. Upton TJ, Hunt PJ and Doogue MP (2014) Hyponatraemic seizure following arginine vasopressin for von Willebrand disease: pernicious, predictable and preventable. *Intern Med J*, 44, 521–522. PMID: 24816315

2. Laffan MA, Lester W, O'Donnell JS, Will A, Tait RC, Goodeve A *et al.* (2014) The diagnosis and management of von Willebrand disease: a United Kingdom Haemophilia Centre Doctors Organization guideline approved by the British Committee for Standards in Haematology. *Br J Haematol*, 167, 453–465. PMID: 25113304

SBA 75 b Chronic eosinophilic leukaemia with *PDGFRB* rearrangement.

In addition to *BCR-ABL1*-positive chronic myeloid leukaemia, imatinib is likely to be effective in patients with myeloid neoplasms with rearrangement of *PDGFRA* or *PDGFRB*.[1,2]

References

1. Bain BJ (2010) Myeloid and lymphoid neoplasms with eosinophilia and abnormalities of *PDGFRA*, *PDGFRB* or *FGFR1*. *Haematologica*, 95, 696–698. PMID: 20442440

2. Apperley J, Gardembas M, Melo J, Russell-Jones R, Bain BJ, Baxter J *et al.* (2002) Response to imatinib mesylate in patients with chronic myeloproliferative diseases with rearrangements of the platelet-derived growth factor receptor beta. *N Engl J Med*, 347, 481–487.

SBA 76 b Ibrutinib.

The features described suggest a diagnosis of chronic lymphocytic leukaemia (CLL). The Bruton's tyrosine kinase (BTK) inhibitor, ibrutinib, is efficacious in this condition.[1,2] Ibrutinib is a B-cell receptor antagonist. Normally signalling through this pathway induces proliferation, apoptosis or anergy but in CLL there is upregulation and constitutive expression of *BTK*, although the gene is not mutated, giving proliferation and survival signals. About 90% of patients show a response to ibrutinib. Mutation of *BTK* can lead to resistance to ibrutinib. Dasatinib has been reported as being efficacious in only a small number of patients.

References

1. Foà R and Guarini A (2013) A mechanism-driven treatment for chronic lymphocytic leukemia? *N Engl J Med*, 369, 85–87. PMID: 23782159
2. Woyach JA, Furman RR, Liu TM, Ozer HG, Zapatka M, Ruppert AS *et al.* (2014) Resistance mechanisms for the Bruton's tyrosine kinase inhibitor ibrutinib. *N Engl J Med*, 370, 2286–2294. PMID: 24869598

SBA 77 b Acute promyelocytic leukaemia

The immunophenotype shows features typical of acute promyelocytic leukaemia.[1,2] The cells are large and the high side scatter is because of their granularity. The lack of expression of CD34, HLA-DR and TdT does not necessarily suggest a chronic myeloid leukaemia, but rather is typical of the promyelocyte stage of maturation and of acute promyelocytic leukaemia. The aberrant expression of CD2 and CD56 is well recognised in this type leukaemia and does not indicate a mixed phenotype. CD9 is often also expressed. CD64 is more typical of monocytic differentiation but is often expressed in acute promyelocytic leukaemia.

References

1. Bain BJ. *Leukaemia Diagnosis*. 4th Edn, Wiley-Blackwell, Oxford, 2010.
2. Leach M, Drummond M and Doig A. *Practical Flow Cytometry in Haematology Diagnosis*. Wiley–Blackwell, Oxford, 2013.

SBA 78 a Arrange magnetic resonance imaging

This serum ferritin measurement would be acceptable in a patient with thalassaemia major. However patients with thalassaemia intermedia have more hepatocyte iron loading relative to macrophage iron than patients with thalassaemia major and this serum ferritin is compatible with significant hepatocyte iron overload. Magnetic resonance imaging should be arranged. In circumstances where this is not available, it is recommended that the serum ferritin be kept below 800 µg/l and that chelation therapy be interrupted when the ferritin falls to 300 µg/l or lower.[1,2]

References

1. Musallam KM, Cappellini MD, Daar S, Karimi M, El-Beshlawy A, Graziadei G et al. (2014) Serum ferritin level and morbidity risk in transfusion-independent patients with β-thalassemia intermedia: the ORIENT study. Haematologica, 99, e218–221. PMID: 24997148
2. Taher AT, Porter JB, Viprakasit V, Kattamis A, Chuncharunee S, Sutcharitchan P et al. (2015) Defining serum ferritin thresholds to predict clinically relevant liver iron concentrations for guiding deferasirox therapy when MRI is unavailable in patients with non-transfusion-dependent thalassaemia. Br J Haematol, 168, 284–290. PMID: 25212456

SBA 79 a Continuation of allopurinol.

The laboratory features indicate tumour lysis syndrome with early signs of acute renal injury.[1,2] Urinary alkalinisation is not indicated since xanthine, hypoxanthine and calcium precipitate in the kidneys in alkaline conditions. Rasburicase should not be administered to someone who is G6PD deficient. Allopurinol and vigorous hydration should be continued, with haemofiltration or haemodialysis being introduced if the situation worsens. Peritoneal dialysis is not indicated since the response is slower.

References

1. Cairo MS, Coiffier B, Reiter A and Younes A; TLS Expert Panel (2010) Recommendations for the evaluation of risk and prophylaxis of tumour lysis syndrome (TLS) in adults and children with malignant diseases: an expert TLS panel consensus. Br J Haematol, 149, 578–586. PMID: 20331465
2. Jones GL, Will A, Jackson GH, Webb N and Rule S (2014) Guidelines for the Management of Tumour Lysis Syndrome in Adults and Children with Haematological Malignancies. Br J Haematol, 169, 661–671. PMID: 2587699

SBA 80 e Solvent detergent-treated fresh frozen plasma.
The features described indicate likely TTP. The only suitable replacement fluid is fresh frozen plasma since it is necessary both to remove high molecular weight von Willebrand factor molecules and anti-ADAMTS13 antibodies and also to replace the deficient ADAMTS13.[1] The plasma should be solvent detergent treated. Gelofusine is an albumin substitute, which can be used for volume expansion.

Reference
1. Scully M, Hunt BJ, Benjamin S, Liesner R, Rose P, Peyvandi F, Cheung B and Machin SJ. On behalf of the British Committee for Standards in Haematology. (2012) Guidelines on the diagnosis and management of thrombotic thrombocytopenic purpura and other thrombotic microangiopathies. *Br J Haematol*, 158, 323–335. PMID: 22624596

SBA 81 d Reduced-intensity treatment.
Results of patients entered into the Medical Research Council UKALL 2003 trial for children, adolescents and young adults with ALL showed that patients with Down syndrome had a higher mortality than other patients with ALL, largely as a result of increased treatment-related mortality.[1] Treatment outcome was improved when less intensive treatment was employed, together with enhanced supportive care.

Reference
1. Patrick K, Wade R, Goulden N, Rowntree C, Hough R, Moorman AV *et al.* (2014) Outcome of Down syndrome associated acute lymphoblastic leukaemia treated on a contemporary protocol. *Br J Haematol*, 165, 552–555. PMID: 24428704

SBA 82 b Aspirin plus low molecular weight heparin.
The evidence base to make an informed choice is not particularly strong. Aspirin plus unfractionated heparin has been found to be associated with a better fetal outcome than aspirin alone (80% versus 40% live birth rate) and two small trials have suggested that aspirin plus low molecular weight heparin is equivalent to aspirin plus unfractionated heparin. Use of unfractionated heparin in pregnancy is generally avoided because of the risk of osteoporosis and haemorrhage. The British Committee for Standards in Haematology (BCSH) advice for a patient such as the one described is that aspirin plus low molecular weight heparin be given.[1]

Reference

1. Keeling D, Mackie I, Moore GW, Greer IA and Greaves M; British Committee for Standards in Haematology (2012) Guidelines on the investigation and management of antiphospholipid syndrome. *Br J Haematol*, 157, 47–58. PMID: 22313321

SBA 83 c *Clostridium perfringens* sepsis.

This case report is derived from the reference given.[1] The features described suggest acute infection by *Clostridium perfringens*. The haemolysis and spherocytosis are due to an exotoxin, which hydrolyses phospholipids in the red cell membrane.

Reference

1. Renaudon-Smith E, Kaur M, Haroon A, Cavenagh J and Butler T (2014) Intravascular haemolysis secondary to Clostridium perfringens in a patient with acute myeloid leukaemia undergoing allogeneic stem cell transplantation. *Br J Haematol*, 165, 743. PMID: 24446867

SBA 84 d A normal thrombin time.

The thrombin time is very sensitive to dabigatran so that a normal thrombin time excludes a clinically significant concentration of the drug.[1] It is not, however, suitable for monitoring therapy.

Reference

1. Kitchen S, Gray E, Mackie I, Baglin T and Makris M (2014) Measurement of non-coumarin anticoagulants and their effects on tests of haemostasis: Guidance from the British Committee for Standards in Haematology. *Br J Haematol*, 166, 830–841. PMID: 24930477

SBA 85 e Rearrangement of *MYC*.

The features described suggest a diagnosis of Burkitt lymphoma. Although BCL6 is expressed the gene is not rearranged. The *MYC* gene is rearranged, usually as a result of t(8;14)(q24;q32). The lymphoma that most often affects the breast is diffuse large B-cell lymphoma. However the immunophenotype and the very high proliferation fraction in this patient are indicative of Burkitt lymphoma, which may be bilateral and may be manifest for the first time during pregnancy or lactation.[1–3] Exceptionally Burkitt lymphoma has presented with simultaneous bilateral tumours of both breast and ovaries.

References

1. Negahban S, Ahmadi N, Oryan A, Khojasteh HN, Aledavood A, Soleimanpour H *et al.* (2010) Primary bilateral Burkitt lymphoma of the lactating breast: a case report and review of the literature. *Mol Diagn Ther*, 14, 243–250. PMID: 20799767
2. Peterson C, Lester DR and Sanger W (2010) Burkitt's lymphoma in early pregnancy. *J Clin Oncol*, 28, e136–138. PMID: 20048180
3. Thieringer F, Sartorius G, Kalf K, Heinzelmann V and Vetter M (2013) Bilateral breast masses with a rare etiology. *Case Rep Oncol Med*, 2013:412368. doi: 10.1155/2013/412368. PMID: 24066248

SBA 86 e Oral corticosteroids.

The features described suggest a diagnosis of autoimmune thrombocytopenic purpura. Although management in children is often conservative, mucosal bleeding is considered an indication for therapy with oral corticosteroids being preferred.[1] The Hb is normal for a child of this age and there is no reason to suspect acute leukaemia.

Reference

1. Cooper N (2014) A review of the management of childhood immune thrombocytopenia: how can we provide an evidence-based approach? *Br J Haematol*, 165, 756–767. PMID: 24761791

SBA 87 b CD1a

The features described suggest a diagnosis of Langerhans cell histiocytosis, not a T-cell or plasma cell neoplasm.[1-3] The neoplastic cells express CD1a and langerin (CD207). Note: this question is more difficult than those usually set in FRCPath examinations but is relevant particularly to paediatric haematologists.

References

1. Badalian-Very G, Vergilio JA, Degar BA, Rodriguez-Galindo C and Rollins BJ (2012) Recent advances in the understanding of Langerhans cell histiocytosis. *Br J Haematol*, 156, 163–172. PMID: 22017623
2. Mehta B and Venkatramani R (2014) Images in clinical medicine. Langerhans'-cell histiocytosis. *N Engl J Med*, 371, 1050. PMID: 25207768
3. Dutta S, Majumder A (2014) A thirsty child. *Blood*, 123, 3854. PMID: 2508352

SBA 88 e Iron-refractory iron deficiency anaemia.

The features are those of iron-refractory iron deficiency anaemia which results from a biallelic mutation in *TMPRSS6*.[1–3] *TMPRSS6* encodes matriptase-2, a membrane serine protease that senses iron deficiency and blocks hepcidin transcription. Mutation leads to failure of inhibition of hepcidin synthesis. High hepcidin concentrations in turn lead to reduced iron absorption and reduced release of iron from macrophages, hence the discrepancy between the normal serum ferritin and the low serum iron and transferrin saturation. Usually there is no response to oral iron but there may be a partial response to parenteral iron.

Note: this question is more difficult than would be expected in the FRC-Path or MRCP examinations.

References

1. Nie N, Shi J, Shao Y, Li X, Ge M, Huang J *et al.* (2014) A novel tri-allelic mutation of TMPRSS6 in iron-refractory iron deficiency anaemia with response to glucocorticoid. *Br J Haematol*, 166, 300–303. PMID: 24661031
2. Camaschella C (2013) How I manage patients with atypical microcytic anaemia. *Br J Haematol*, 160, 12–24. PMID: 23057559
3. Donker AE, Raymakers RA, Vlasveld LT, van Barneveld T, Terink R, Dors N *et al.* (2014) Practice guidelines for the diagnosis and management of microcytic anemias due to genetic disorders of iron metabolism or heme synthesis. *Blood*, 123, 3873–3886. PMID: 24665134

SBA 89 c Phlebotomy to normalise iron stores.

Although it is counter-intuitive, it is recommended that iron stores should be normalised by cautious phlebotomy prior to commencing pyridoxine therapy.[1,2] This can actually lead to an increase in Hb since mitochondrial iron loading exacerbates the anaemia by reducing pyridoxine sensitivity. Once iron stores are normalised, pyridoxine can be commenced in a dose of 50–200 mg, with the dose being lowered once a response has occurred.

References

1. Cotter PD, May A, Li L, Al-Sabah AI, Fitzsimons EJ, Cazzola M and Bishop DF (1999) Four new mutations in the erythroid-specific 5-aminolevulinate synthase (ALAS2) gene causing X-linked sideroblastic anemia: increased pyridoxine responsiveness after removal of iron overload by phlebotomy and coinheritance of hereditary hemochromatosis. *Blood*, 93, 1757–1769. PMID: 10029606

2. Donker AE, Raymakers RA, Vlasveld LT, van Barneveld T, Terink R, Dors N *et al.* (2014) Practice guidelines for the diagnosis and management of microcytic anemias due to genetic disorders of iron metabolism or heme synthesis. *Blood*, 123, 3873–3886. PMID: 24665134

SBA 90 a Cautious paracentesis and defibrotide.

The features described suggest severe sinusoidal obstruction syndrome (previously known as hepatic veno-occlusive disease). Sirolimus and conditioning with busulphan are risk factors and in fact the use of sirolimus after busulphan conditioning is not recommended.[1-3] Diuretics and paracentesis should be used only cautiously in sinusoidal obstruction syndrome as renal blood flow may otherwise be reduced leading to hepatorenal syndrome. For severe cases, defibrotide to induce fibrinolysis appears to be of benefit, when treatment results are compared with historical controls. Tissue plasminogen activator and heparin are not recommended because of the risk of haemorrhage. Since this patient has respiratory distress, paracentesis is also indicated but the volume of ascitic fluid removed should be restricted to about a litre a day.

References

1. Cutler C, Stevenson K, Kim HT, Richardson P, Ho VT, Linden E *et al.* (2008) Sirolimus is associated with veno-occlusive disease of the liver after myeloablative allogeneic stem cell transplantation. *Blood*, 112, 4425–1431. PMID: 18776081
2. Dignan FL, Wynn RF, Hadzic N, Karani J, Quaglia A, Pagliuca A *et al.*; Haemato-oncology Task Force of British Committee for Standards in Haematology; British Society for Blood and Marrow Transplantation (2013) BCSH/BSBMT guideline: diagnosis and management of veno-occlusive disease (sinusoidal obstruction syndrome) following haematopoietic stem cell transplantation. *Br J Haematol*, 163, 444–457. PMID: 24102514
3. Chao N (2014) How I treat sinusoidal obstruction syndrome. *Blood*, 123, 4023–4026. PMID: 24833355

SBA 91 e Is increased leading to impaired release of iron from macrophages and reduced delivery of iron into the plasma by enterocytes.

Hepcidin is synthesised by hepatocytes. Synthesis is increased in inflammation as a result of increased interleukin 6. This leads to impaired release of iron from enterocytes into the plasma, impaired delivery of iron from macrophages and reduced mobilisation of hepatocyte iron.[1] As a result, the plasma iron falls and inadequate iron is available for haemoglobin synthesis.

Reference

1. Kautz L and Nemeth E (2014) Molecular liaisons between erythropoiesis and iron metabolism. *Blood*, 124, 479–482. PMID: 24876565

SBA 92 b High dose methotrexate followed by dose-intensive consolidation chemotherapy

Whole brain irradiation is not indicated since although the early response is good, neurocognitive impairment occurs and survival is poor. Best results are obtained with high dose methotrexate followed by dose-intensive consolidation chemotherapy, this yielding median progression-free survival of 2 years and an expected overall survival of 40–50%.[1,2]

References

1. Wang CC, Carnevale J and Rubenstein JL (2014) Progress in central nervous system lymphomas. *Br J Haematol*, 166, 311–325. PMID: 24837460
2. Plotkin SR and Batchelor TT (2001) Primary nervous-system lymphoma. *Lancet Oncol*, 2, 354–365. PMID: 11905752

SBA 93 b Chromogenic assay for anti-thrombin activity.

Dabigatran is a direct-acting anti-thrombin, which does not usually require monitoring. However testing is relevant when a patient has suffered a haemorrhage. A chromogenic assay of antithrombin activity with a dabigatran-specific calibrator is recommended.[1] Alternatives would be a modified thrombin time with a dabigatran-specific calibrator or an ecarin clotting time. An APTT cannot be used for judging drug concentration as the relationship is curvilinear. A normal thrombin time suggests that the level of dabigatran is likely to be very low.

Reference

1. Kitchen S, Gray E, Mackie I, Baglin T and Makris M; BCSH committee (2014) Measurement of non-coumarin anticoagulants and their effects on tests of haemostasis: Guidance from the British Committee for Standards in Haematology. *Br J Haematol*, 166, 830–841. PMID: 24930477

SBA 94 a Copper deficiency.

The clinical and haematological features are those of copper deficiency, for which bariatric surgery is a well recognised cause.[1,2] Although vitamin B_{12} could cause these neurological features and a macrocytic anaemia, it would not cause disproportionate neutropenia and vacuolation of haemopoietic precursors.

References
1. Chhetri SK, Mills RJ, Shaunak S and Emsley HC (2014) Copper deficiency. *BMJ*, 348, 37–39. PMID: 24938531
2. Mangles SE, Abdalla SH, Gabriel CM and Bain B (2007) Case Report 37: Neutropenia and macrocytosis in a middle-aged man. *Leuk Lymphoma*, 48, 1846–1848. PMID: 17786722

SBA 95 d Heterozygosity for either β thalassaemia or haemoglobin S.

The diagnosis in the young woman is haemoglobin S/β⁺ thalassaemia compound heterozygosity. Of relevance in her partner would be β thalassaemia heterozygosity (with a risk of either β thalassaemia major or haemoglobin S/β thalassaemia compound heterozygosity in the fetus) or haemoglobin S (risk of sickle cell anaemia or haemoglobin S/β thalassaemia compound heterozygosity in the fetus). There is no reason to suspect an underlying α thalassaemia so neither α⁰ thalassaemia heterozygosity nor haemoglobin H disease would be relevant. Note that both haemoglobin S and β thalassaemia occur in Sicily. β thalassaemia is highly prevalent and haemoglobin S heterozygosity occurs in about 2% of Sicilians.[1]

Reference
1. Russo G and Schiliro G (2014) Sickle cell anemia and S-thalassemia in Sicilian children. http://sicklecellsociety.org/resources/sickle-cell-anemia-in-sicilian-children/ (accessed February 2015)

SBA 96 b Haemopoietic stem cell transplantation.

The clinicopathological features are indicative of juvenile myelomonocytic leukaemia. This child has bad prognostic features (age over 4 years, haemoglobin F over 40% and platelet count less than 33×10^9/l).[1] Early haemopoietic stem cell transplantation is indicated. In this patient there is no specific indication for chemotherapy, which might be considered if there were a high white cell count, marked hepatosplenomegaly or respiratory symptoms.

Reference
1. Chang TY, Dvorak CC and Loh ML (2014) Bedside to bench in juvenile myelomonocytic leukemia: insights into leukemogenesis from a rare pediatric leukemia. *Blood*, 124, 2487–2497. PMID: 25163700

SBA 97 b Danazol.
The patient has post-polycythaemia myelofibrosis. As the serum erythropoietin is high, neither erythropoietin nor darbepoetin would be likely to be of benefit whereas danazol may well be useful.[1] Ruxolitinib is not of benefit for anaemia.

Reference
1. Cervantes F (2014) How I treat myelofibrosis. *Blood*, 124, 2635–2642. PMID: 25232060

SBA 98 b DNA analysis for α^0 thalassaemia.
The haemoglobin E plus A_2 percentage is considerably less than would be expected in a haemoglobin E heterozygote and suggests that she may also be heterozygous for α^0 thalassaemia (or homozygous for α^+ thalassaemia).[1] DNA analysis would therefore be a reasonable action. An alternative would be to test her partner and only perform DNA analysis if he had a relevant haematological abnormality. Capillary electrophoresis would permit the quantification of haemoglobin A_2 and haemoglobin E but would not advance the diagnosis. Iron deficiency would not account for marked microcytosis with only a slight reduction of Hb so serum ferritin is unlikely to be helpful.

Reference
1. Pornprasert S, Treesuwan K, Punyamung M and Kongthai K (2012) Hb A_2/E levels found in co-inheritance with the α-thalassemia-1 - -[SEA]/type deletion and either Hb E or β-thalassemia. *Hemoglobin*, 36, 381–387. PMID: 22563848

SBA 99 c β thalassaemia heterozygosity.

It is important to realise that haemoglobin E homozygosity is generally an asymptomatic condition whereas compound heterozygosity for haemoglobin E and β thalassaemia is a potentially serious condition that may have the phenotype of thalassaemia intermedia or major.[1] There is no reason to suspect α^0 thalassaemia in the patient since this degree of microcytosis is expected in haemoglobin E heterozygosity and if there were co-existing α thalassaemia the haemoglobin percentage would be likely to be lower. The suspicion of α thalassaemia in the partner would therefore not be a cause for concern.

Reference

1. Winichagoon P, Thonglairoam V, Fucharoen S, Wilairat P, Fukumaki Y and Wasi P (1993) Severity differences in β-thalassaemia/haemoglobin E syndromes: implication of genetic factors. *Br J Haematol*, 83, 633–639.

SBA 100 a Intrinsic factor antibodies.

The diagnosis you should suspect is pernicious anaemia in view of the macrocytic anaemia and the history of hypothyroidism. Of the tests listed, a test for intrinsic factor antibodies is the most specific, although parietal cell antibodies, serum vitamin B_{12} and serum holotranscobalamin assay would be more sensitive.[1]

Reference

1. Harrington D. Investigation of megaloblastic anaemia: cobalamin, folate and metabolite status. *In* Bain BJ, Bates I and Laffan MA (Eds) *Dacie and Lewis Practical Haematology* 12th Edn, Churchill–Livingstone, 2016.

SBA 101 c Less than 5 days old, CMV-negative, taken into citrate-phosphate-dextrose (CPD), irradiated.

Blood for use for neonatal exchange transfusion should be:

a. Less than 5 days old, to reduce the risk of hyperkalaemia
b. Negative for high titre anti-A and anti-B antibodies.
c. Taken into CPD rather than SAG-M (saline, adenine, glucose, mannitol), to reduce the potential risk of toxicity from adenine or mannitol

d. CMV-negative
e. Irradiated (to prevent graft-versus host disease)
f. With a haematocrit of 0.50–0.60 (to reduce the risk of post-procedure anaemia or polycythaemia).[1]

Reference
1. Transfusion guidelines for neonates and older children http://onlinelibrary.wiley.com/doi/10.1111/j.1365-2141.2004.04815.x/full (accessed November 2015)

SBA 102 d POEMS syndrome.

The constellation of abnormalities described is indicative of the POEMS syndrome, indicating Polyneuropathy, Organomegaly (hepatomegaly, splenomegaly, lymphadenopathy), Endocrinopathy, M-protein and Skin changes.[1] A diagnosis of solitary plasmacytoma would be less appropriate, there is not enough evidence for a diagnosis of multiple myeloma and, given the presence of the plasmacytoma, a diagnosis of MGUS would be wrong. The POEMS syndrome results from an underlying plasma cell neoplasm with the unusual range of clinicopathological features thought to result from secretion of cytokines such as vascular endothelial growth factor (VEGF) and interleukin 12.

Reference
1. Smith C, Saint S, Price R, Al-Zoubi A and Callaghan B (2015) Clinical problem-solving. Diagnosing one letter at a time. *N Engl J Med*, 372, 67–73. PMID: 25551528

SBA 103 b Aspirin, venesection and hydroxycarbamide.

There is enough evidence for a diagnosis of polycythaemia vera (of the WHO criteria, one major and two minor criteria are met). Because of his age and previous vascular event the patient falls into a high risk group.[1] He therefore need cytoreduction in addition to aspirin. It would be prudent to lower the Hct by venesection while waiting for hydroxycarbamide to take effect.

Reference
1. Vannucchi AM (2014) How I treat polycythemia vera. *Blood*, 124, 3212–3220. PMID: 25278584

SBA 104 c Observation.

The diagnosis is transient abnormal myelopoiesis of Down syndrome, not acute leukaemia.[1,2] There is not currently any need for red cell or platelet transfusion. There is certainly no indication for chemotherapy, which would only be appropriate if the WBC were very high with a risk of leucostasis. A spontaneous remission is expected although about a quarter of such babies go on to develop AML a few years later.

References
1. Roberts I and Izraeli S (2014) Haematopoietic development and leukaemia in Down syndrome. *Br J Haematol*, 167, 587–599. PMID: 25155832
2. Litz CE, Davies S, Brunning RD, Kueck B, Parkin JL, Gajl Peczalska K and Arthur DC (1995) Acute leukemia and the transient myeloproliferative disorder associated with Down syndrome: morphologic, immunophenotypic and cytogenetic manifestations. *Leukemia*, 9, 1432–1439. PMID: 7658708

SBA 105 b Normal for age.

Anti-A and anti-B are not expected in a baby of this age. The baby has mild polycythaemia as a result of the cyanotic heart disease but otherwise the blood count is normal for age. There is no reason to suspect any immunological abnormality. Note that maternal plasma should be screened for atypical antibodies. There may have been transplacental passage of antibodies, which are present at a higher titre and more readily detectable in maternal plasma than in the infant's plasma.

SBA 106 c Intravenous methylene blue.

Intravenous methylene blue is very effective treatment in methaemoglobinaemia, except in patients who are G6PD deficient.[1,2] As the patient has been identified as female and Northern European Caucasian, testing for G6PD deficiency is not necessary. Methaemoglobinaemia is a recognised feature of oral dapsone therapy. Rarely it has followed use of topical dapsone.[2]

References
1. Sikka P, Bindra VK, Kapoor S, Jain V and Saxena KK (2011) Blue cures blue but be cautious. *J Pharm Bioallied Sci*, 3, 543–545. PMID: 22219589

2. Swartzentruber GS, Yanta JH and Pizon AF (2015) Methemoglobinemia as a complication of topical dapsone. *N Engl J Med*, 372, 491–492. PMID: 25629756

SBA 107 c Commencement of argatroban and administration of vitamin K.

Fondaparinux has been used with success in the treatment of HIT but since it has been responsible for a small number of cases of HIT, a non-heparin anticoagulant such as argatroban is preferred.[1] There has also been a report of failure of the platelet count to improve, due to cross-reacting antibodies, when a patient with HIT was switched to fondaparinux.[2] If a vitamin K antagonist has been started, its effects should be reversed since protein C levels fall more rapidly than prothrombin levels and, in patients with HIT, venous gangrene can occur. Low molecular weight heparin is contraindicated.

References
1. Linkins LA (2015) Heparin induced thrombocytopenia. *BMJ*, 350, 27–30. PMID: 25569604
2. Creasey T, Murphy P and Talks K (2015) A case of heparin-induced thrombocytopenia with thrombosis and cross-reacting antibodies successfully treated with rivaroxaban. *Br J Haematol*, 169, Suppl. 1, 44–45.

SBA 108 a Compound heterozygosity for β⁰ thalassaemia and δβ thalassaemia.

The baby's father has β thalassaemia heterozygosity. Her mother has both microcytosis and an increased haemoglobin F so her diagnosis is δβ thalassaemia rather than hereditary persistence of fetal haemoglobin. The baby has thalassaemia major and has no haemoglobin A. We can therefore deduce that she must have compound heterozygosity for β⁰ thalassaemia and δβ thalassaemia and the thalassaemia trait in her father must be β⁰ thalassaemia trait not β⁺ thalassaemia trait.[1]

Reference
1. Mann JR, Macneish AS, Bannister D, Clegg JB, Wood WG and Weatherall DJ (1972) δβ-thalassaemia in a Chinese family. *Br J Haematol*, 23, 393–402. PMID: 5084805

SBA 109 c Continue warfarin at the same dose as long as the INR is in the therapeutic range.

Cataract surgery has a low risk of haemorrhage and no alteration of his treatment is indicated.

SBA 110 b Herpes zoster.

Although the incidence of herpes zoster is considerably increased in chronic lymphocytic leukaemia (CLL), it is very important NOT to administer herpes zoster vaccine to a significantly immunosuppressed patient.[1] You should be aware that in the UK this vaccine is usually administered at the age of 70 years so the patient and his GP should be made aware that he should not receive it. There is no contra-indication to the other vaccines listed.

Reference
1. https://www.gov.uk/government/collections/immunisation-against-infectious-disease-the-green-book (accessed April 2015)

SBA 111 d Haemoglobin D-Punjab trait.

Neither α^0 thalassaemia nor haemoglobin G-Philadelphia trait will interact adversely with haemoglobin S trait. Haemoglobin D-Punjab is of most relevance since the compound heterozygous state with haemoglobin S has a severe phenotype. An interaction with haemoglobin E or hereditary persistence of fetal haemoglobin causes only a mild disorder, if any.[1,2]

References
1. Sickle Cell and Thalassaemia: Handbook for Laboratories. http://sct.screening.nhs.uk/standardsandguidelines (accessed April 2015)
2. Bain BJ, Wild BJ, Stephens AD and Phelan LA. *Variant Haemoglobins: a Guide to Identification.* Wiley-Blackwell, Oxford, 2010.

SBA 112 e Ruxolitinib.

The patient's disease control is inadequate. Ruxolitinib is generally successful in treating polycythaemia vera patients who are refractory to hydroxycarbamide or intolerant of it. It lowers the haematocrit, reduces splenomegaly, ameliorates symptoms and reduces the burden of the V617F mutant *JAK2* allele[1]. Busulphan, pipobroman and ^{32}P are all thought to be leukaemogenic. Interferon can be efficacious but is often not tolerated.

Reference
1. Vannucchi AM, Kiladjian JJ, Griesshammer M, Masszi T, Durrant S, Passamonti F *et al.* (2015) Ruxolitinib versus standard therapy for the treatment of polycythemia vera. *N Engl J Med*, 372, 426–435. PMID: 25629741

SBA 113 e Rituximab in a dose of 375 mg/m^2 weekly for 4 weeks.

The patient has refractory autoimmune haemolytic anaemia (AIHA) and already has corticosteroid side effects so an increase in dose would be unwise. Second line treatment is now rituximab rather than splenectomy. The response rate is high[1] and the risk of complications less. Alemtuzumab and mycophenolate mofetil are third line rather than second line treatment options.

Reference
1. Maung SW, Leahy M, O'Leary HM, Khan I, Cahill MR, Gilligan O *et al.* (2013) A multi-centre retrospective study of rituximab use in the treatment of relapsed or resistant warm autoimmune haemolytic anaemia. *Br J Haematol*, 163, 118–122. PMID: 23909468

SBA 114 c Hyperdiploidy.
Hyperdiploidy is associated with a standard prognosis in multiple myeloma. The other cytogenetic and molecular abnormalities are associated with a worse prognosis.[1–3]

References
1. Rajkumar SV (2013) Multiple myeloma: 2013 update on diagnosis, risk-stratification, and management. *Am J Hematol*, 88, 226–235. PMID: 23440663
2. Pratt G, Jenner M, Owen R, Snowden JA, Ashcroft J, Yong K *et al.* (2014) Updates to the guidelines for the diagnosis and management of multiple myeloma. *Br J Haematol*, 167, 131–133. PMID: 24801672

3. Rajkumar SV, Dimopoulos MA, Palumbo A, Blade J, Merlini G, Mateos MV *et al.* (2014) International Myeloma Working Group updated criteria for the diagnosis of multiple myeloma. *Lancet Oncol*, 15, e538–548. PMID: 25439696

SBA 115 e Hereditary xerocytosis.

The findings are those of hereditary xerocytosis, also known as the dehydrated form of hereditary stomatocytosis.[1,2] Leaking of potassium from red cells causing pseudohyperkalaemia can be a feature.[2] Exercise-induced haemolysis has been described.[1]

References
1. Archer NM, Shmukler BE, Andolfo I, Vandorpe DH, Gnanasambandam R, Higgins JM *et al.* (2014) Hereditary xerocytosis revisited. *Am J Hematol*, 89, 1142–1146. PMID: 25044010
2. Gore DM, Layton M, Sinha AK, Williamson PJ, Vaidya B, Connolly V *et al.* (2004) Four pedigrees of the cation-leaky hereditary stomatocytosis class presenting with pseudohyperkalaemia. Novel profile of temperature dependence of Na+-K+ leak in xerocytic form. *Br J Haematol*, 125, 521–527. PMID: 15142123

SBA 116 a BCR-ABL1.

The megakaryocyte morphology indicates that this is likely to be a variant of chronic myelogenous leukaemia (CML) with *BCR-ABL1*. The other mutations are associated with myeloproliferative neoplasms but not with small, hypolobated megakaryocytes. This condition is sometimes designated Ph-positive essential thrombocythaemia (ET) but in the WHO classification it is appropriately categorised as a variant of CML rather than of ET.[1]

Reference
1. Vardiman J, Melo JV, Baccarani M and Thiele J. Chronic myelogenous leukaemia, *BCR-ABL1* positive. *In* Swerdlow SH, Campo E, Harris NL, Jaffe ES, Pileri SA, Stein H, Thiele J and Vardiman JW, *World Health Organization Classification of Tumours of Haematopoietic and Lymphoid Tissues*, 4th Edn, IARC Press, Lyon, 2008, pp 32–37.

SBA 117 e Intensive combination chemotherapy plus rituximab plus HAART.

Optimal management is combination immunochemotherapy plus highly active anti-retroviral therapy (HAART).[1,2] This is associated with an improved complete remission rate in comparison with alternatives. Although rituximab lowers serum immunoglobulin, its inclusion is associated with an improved overall survival, at least in those with a CD4 lymphocyte count above $100/mm^3$. Superior outcome has been observed with more intensive regimes, such as EPOCH and ACVBP, in comparison with CHOP.

References

1. Barta SK, Xue X, Wang D, Tamari R, Lee JY, Mounier N *et al.* (2013) Treatment factors affecting outcomes in HIV-associated non-Hodgkin lymphomas: a pooled analysis of 1546 patients. *Blood*, 122, 3251–3262. PMID: 24014242
2. Levine AM (2013) AIDS-lymphoma (ARL): one more step along the way. *Blood*, 122, 3244–3246. PMID: 24203926

SBA 118 d This variant haemoglobin can interact adversely with haemoglobin S and β thalassaemia.

Despite its name, haemoglobin O-Arab is not particularly common in Arabs. It has been identified also in Greeks, Turks, Eastern Europeans and North and East Africans. Compound heterozygosity with haemoglobin S causes a severe form of sickle cell disease, while interaction with β thalassaemia can cause thalassaemia intermedia. Although antenatal diagnosis should be carried out as early in pregnancy as possible, investigation at 16 weeks gestation is still justified.

Reference

1. Bain BJ, Wild BJ, Stephens AD and Phelan LA. *Variant Haemoglobins: a Guide to Identification.* Wiley-Blackwell, Oxford, 2010.

SBA 119 e Neutrophilic leukaemoid reaction.

The presence of a paraprotein in high concentration indicates that the patient has multiple myeloma. It is therefore very likely that the patient has a neutrophilic leukaemoid reaction mediated by granulocyte colony-stimulating factor secreted by the myeloma cells.[1] It should be noted that toxic granulation and Döhle bodies can also be seen in chronic neutrophilic leukaemia but a coincidental association of chronic neutrophilic leukaemia and multiple myeloma is much less common than a leukaemoid reaction to myeloma.

Reference

1. Bain BJ and Ahmad S (2015) Chronic neutrophilic leukaemia and plasma cell-related neutrophilic leukaemoid reactions. *Br J Haematol*, 171, 400–410.

SBA 120 d Persistent polyclonal B lymphocytosis.

These distinctive cytological features are characteristic of persistent polyclonal B lymphocytosis, a condition that typically occurs in female cigarette smokers.[1] It is associated with HLA-DR7 and familial cases have been reported.

Reference

1. Deplano S, Nadal-Melsió E and Bain BJ (2014) Persistent polyclonal B lymphocytosis. *Am J Hematol*, 89, 224. PMID: 24227021

Section 5:
Extended Matching Questions
Answers and Feedback

Multiple Choice Questions for Haematology and Core Medical Trainees, First Edition.
Barbara J. Bain.
© 2016 John Wiley & Sons, Ltd. Published 2016 by John Wiley & Sons, Ltd.

EMQ 1

(i) j T-cell prolymphocytic leukaemia. This is a fairly typical case.[1–3]

(ii) d Angioimmunoblastic T-cell lymphoma. The immunophenotype is typical with T cells expressing CD10 and CD279 (a marker of follicular helper T cells).[4]

(iii) f Extranodal NK/T-cell lymphoma, nasal type. This condition is Epstein–Barr virus (EBV) related and is more common in Chinese and Central and South American populations. Most cases have the markers of natural killer (NK) cells. These cases may express CD3ε, detectable with polyclonal antibodies, but not surface membrane CD3.

(iv) a Adult T-cell leukaemia/lymphoma. This patient has hypercalcaemia and an immunophenotype compatible with this condition.[5]

(v) i T-cell precursor lymphoblastic leukaemia/lymphoma. There is an immature phenotype with co-expression of CD4 and CD8, typical of precursor-T lymphoblastic leukaemia/lymphoma (T-lineage acute lymphoblastic leukaemia). Note that CD7 is expressed whereas in lymphomas of mature T-cells, with the exception of T-prolymphocytic leukaemia, CD7 is often not expressed.

References

1. Paul RN, Alizadeh L, Ajayi OI, Karpurapu H, Ganesan C, Taddesse-Heath L and Aggarwal A (2012) A case report of T cell prolymphocytic leukemia and Kaposi sarcoma and a review of T cell prolymphocytic leukemia. *Acta Haematol*, 127, 235–243. PMID: 22517037
2. Parker A, Bain B, Devereux S, Gatter K, Jack A, Matutes E *et al*. British Committee for Standards in Haematology (2010) Best Practice in Lymphoma Diagnosis and Reporting. http://www.bcshguidelines.com/documents/Lymphoma_diagnosis_bcsh_042010.pdf (accessed April 2015)
3. Parker A, Bain B, Devereux S, Gatter K, Jack A, Matutes E *et al*. British Committee for Standards in Haematology (2010) Best Practice in Lymphoma Diagnosis and Reporting: specific disease appendix. http://www.bcshguidelines.com/documents/Lymphoma_disease_app_bcsh_042010.pdf (accessed April 2015)
4. Smeltzer JP, Viswanatha DS, Habermann TM and Patnaik MM (2012) Secondary Epstein-Barr virus associated lymphoproliferative disorder developing in a patient with angioimmunoblastic T cell lymphoma on vorinostat. *Am J Hematol*, 87, 927–928. PMID: 22718468
5. Fathi AT, Chen YB, Carter BW and Ryan RJ (2012) Case records of the Massachusetts General Hospital. Case 24-2012. A 38-year-old man with abdominal pain and altered mental status. *N Engl J Med*, 367, 552–563. PMID: 22873536

EMQ 2

(i) c Fibrinogen concentrate. Fibrinogen concentrate is preferred to pathogen-reduced cryoprecipitate, particularly in this grave situation.[1]

(ii) g Recombinant activated factor VII. This is the preferred blood product but if it is unavailable, plasma-derived factor VII is an alternative.[1]

(iii) j Tranexamic acid. This patient could be managed in the first instance by local measures plus tranexamic acid. There is a poor correlation between bleeding manifestations and factor levels in factor XI deficiency.[1]

(iv) i Solvent-detergent-treated fresh frozen plasma. For major surgery this is the product currently available and required. A factor V concentrate is under development.[1]

(v) b Factor XI concentrate. This patient has had a significant haemorrhage and factor XI concentrate is indicated. There are two unlicensed products available. Solvent-detergent-treated fresh frozen plasma would be an alternative if the factor concentrate were not available.[1]

Reference

1. Mumford AA, Ackroyd S, Alikhan R, Bowles L, Chowdary P, Grainger J et al. BCSH (2014) Guideline for the diagnosis and management of the rare coagulation disorders: a United Kingdom Haemophilia Centre Doctors' Organization guideline on behalf of the British Committee for Standards in Haematology. *Br J Haematol*, 167, 304–326. PMID: 25100430

EMQ 3

(i) g Transfusion-associated acute lung injury (TRALI). TRALI is most common after plasma transfusion followed by platelet transfusion then red cell transfusion.[1,2]

(ii) a Acute haemolytic transfusion reaction. ABO incompatibility is still the most common cause of an acute haemolytic transfusion reaction. Less often it is due to other antibodies that can bind complement, such as anti-Jka.[2]

(iii) b Anaphylactic transfusion reaction. Anaphylactic transfusion reactions are most often due to anti-immunoglobulin (Ig) A antibodies. Less often they result from a reaction to a foreign antigen present in donor blood, for example, peanut antigens.[2]

(iv) f Septic transfusion reaction. Because of their storage at room temperature, platelet concentrates remain the most common cause of septic transfusion reactions.[2]

(v) c Delayed haemolytic transfusion reaction. Delayed transfusion reactions usually result from transfusion of red cells expressing an antigen to which the patient was previously immunised by transfusion or pregnancy but with the antibody responsible having dropped to an undetectable level.[2]

References

1. Vlaar AP and Juffermans NP (2013) Transfusion-related acute lung injury: a clinical review. *Lancet*, 382, 984–994. PMID: 23642914
2. Torres R, Kenney and Tormey CA (2012) Diagnosis, treatment, and reporting of adverse effects of transfusion. *Lab Med*, 43, 217–231.

EMQ 4

(i) e Drug-induced microangiopathy, immune. Quinine is a well documented cause of immune drug-induced microangiopathy.[1,2]

(ii) j Thrombotic thrombocytopenic purpura (TTP). An ADAMTS13 of less than 10% is a very useful diagnostic feature in TTP.[1,2]

(iii) d Drug-induced microangiopathy, dose-related. This is a recognised dose-related toxicity of tacrolimus.[1,2]

(iv) f Haemolytic uraemic syndrome. One might suspect that the school trip was to a farm or that the child has eaten contaminated food. However, it should be noted that farms now make strenuous efforts to encourage visitors to wash their hands after touching animals.[1,2]

(v) h Hereditary thrombotic thrombocytopenic purpura. A congenital deficiency of ADAMTS13 should be suspected. Patients can present in the neonatal period. Cobalamin C deficiency can also cause microangiopathy but the features described are more consistent with congenital ADAMTS13 deficiency.[1,2]

References

1. George JN and Nester CM (2014) Syndromes of thrombotic microangiopathy. *N Engl J Med*, 371, 654–666. PMID: 25119611
2. Crawley JT and Scully MA (2013) Thrombotic thrombocytopenic purpura: basic pathophysiology and therapeutic strategies. *Hematology Am Soc Hematol Educ Program* 2013, 292–299. PMID: 24319194 http://asheducationbook.hematologylibrary.org/content/2013/1/292.long (accessed June 2015)

EMQ 5

(i) f *MYH9*-related disease. The bilateral sensorineural deafness in combination with familial macrothrombocytopenia is indicative of *MYH9*-related disease. This case might previously have been classified as Epstein syndrome. Although neutrophil inclusions were not identified by light microscopy they were demonstrated by immunofluorescence.[1]

(ii) c Bernard–Soulier syndrome. The severity of the bleeding with a platelet count of 36×10^9/l indicates that the previous diagnosis of autoimmune thrombocytopenic purpura is likely to have been wrong. Bernard–Soulier syndrome is a more likely diagnosis.

(iii) a Alloimmune thrombocytopenia. The most likely explanation is that the mother has antibodies against fetal platelet antigens. Most often these are directed at anti-HPA-1a and less often anti-HPA-5b.[2]

(iv) f *MYH9*-related disease. This is another example of *MYH9*-related disease, specifically May–Hegglin anomaly.

(v) j Wiskott–Aldrich syndrome. Thrombocytopenia with small platelets, eczema and immune deficiency suggest this syndrome.

References

1. Kunishima S, Matsushita T, Shiratsuchi M, Ikuta T, Nishimura J, Hamaguchi M *et al.* (2005) Detection of unique neutrophil non-muscle myosin heavy chain-A localization by immunofluorescence analysis in MYH9 disorder presented with macrothrombocytopenia without leukocyte inclusions and deafness. *Eur J Haematol*, 74, 1–5. PMID: 15613099
2. Murphy MF and Williamson LM (2000) Antenatal screening for fetomaternal alloimmune thrombocytopenia: an evaluation using the criteria of the UK National Screening Committee. *Br J Haematol*, 111, 726–732. PMID: 11122131

EMQ 6

(i) j Two courses of ABVD followed by 20 Gy radiotherapy. Trials have shown that for early stage favourable disease combined modality therapy is superior to radiotherapy alone. Two courses of ABVD followed by 20 Gy radiotherapy is sufficient. ABVD alone may be a suitable option but is associated with a higher relapse rate.[1,2]

(ii) c Four courses of ABVD followed by 30 Gy radiotherapy. This patient has unfavourable stage IIb disease so needs more intensive treatment than the first patient. Four courses of ABVD followed by 30 Gy radiotherapy is therefore appropriate.[1]

(iii) h Six courses of either ABVD or escalated BEACOPP. This patient has stage IIIB disease and either ABVD or escalated BEACOPP would be suitable. BEACOPP has an advantage with regard to progression-free survival but no clear advantage with regard to overall survival and is more toxic.[1]

(iv) g Six courses of ABVD. Escalated BEACOPP is not advised in patients over the age of 60 years so this patient should have ABVD.[1]

(v) a Antiretroviral therapy plus six cycles of ABVD. Escalated BEACOPP is not established treatment in HIV-positive patients so this patient should have antiretroviral treatment plus ABVD.[1]

References

1. Follows GA, Ardeshna KM, Barrington SF, Culligan DJ, Hoskin PJ, Linch D et al. (Writing Group) on behalf of the British Committee for Standards in Haematology (2014) Guidelines for the first line management of classical Hodgkin lymphoma. *Br J Haematol*, 166, 34–49. PMID: 24712411
2. Engert, A., J. Franklin, Eich HT, Brillant C, Sehlen S, Cartoni C et al. (2007) Two cycles of doxorubicin, bleomycin, vinblastine, and dacarbazine plus extended-field radiotherapy is superior to radiotherapy alone in early favorable Hodgkin's lymphoma: final results of the GHSG HD7 trial. *J Clin Oncol*, 25, 3495–3502. PMID: 17606976

EMQ 7

(i) e Epstein–Barr virus. HIV-associated intracerebral diffuse large B-cell lymphoma is very strongly linked to the Epstein–Barr virus.[1]

(ii) g *Helicobacter heilmannii.* Gastric MALT-type lymphoma is strongly linked to *H. pylori* infection but cases have also occurred with *H. heilmannii* and are similarly responsive to antibiotic therapy.[2]

(iii) i Hepatitis C. Marginal zone lymphoma is linked to hepatitis C infection and may respond to antiviral treatment with interferon with or without ribavirin.[3]

(iv) d *Chlamydophila psittaci. Chlamydophila psittaci* (previously *Chlamydia psittaci*) is linked to ocular adnexal MALT-type lymphoma.[4]

(v) b *Borrelia burgdorferi.* Cutaneous MALT-type lymphoma is linked to infection with *Borrelia burgdorferi*, the causative organism of Lyme disease.[5]

References

1. Singh NN (2013) Central nervous system lymphoma in HIV. http://emedicine.medscape.com/article/1167482-overview (accessed June 2015)
2. Morgner A, Lehn N, Andersen LP, Thiede C, Bennedsen M, Trebesius K *et al.* (2000) Helicobacter heilmannii-associated primary gastric low-grade MALT lymphoma: complete remission after curing the infection. *Gastroenterology*, 118, 821–828. PMID: 10784580
3. Arcaini L, Merli M, Volpetti S, Rattotti S, Gotti M and Zaja F (2012) Indolent B-cell lymphomas associated with HCV infection: clinical and virological features and role of antiviral therapy. *Clin Dev Immunol*, 2012:638185. doi: 10.1155/2012/638185
4. Collina F, De Chiara A, De Renzo A, De Rosa G, Botti G and Franco R (2012) Chlamydia psittaci in ocular adnexa MALT lymphoma: a possible role in lymphomagenesis and a different geographical distribution. *Infect Agent Cancer*, 7, 8. PMID: 22472082
5. Goodlad JR, Davidson MM, Hollowood K, Batstone P and Ho-Yen DO (2000) Primary cutaneous B-cell lymphoma and Borrelia burgdorferi infection in patients from the Highlands of Scotland. *Histopathology*, 37, 501–508. PMID: 11122431

EMQ 8

(i) h Iron deficiency anaemia. A low serum iron by itself is of little diagnostic value but when coupled with a high transferrin or total iron binding capacity is indicative of iron deficiency anaemia.[1]

(ii) c β thalassaemia heterozygosity. The FBC is typical of thalassaemia and the elevated haemoglobin A_2 shows that this is β thalassaemia heterozygosity.[2]

(iii) i Iron deficiency plus anaemia of chronic disease. There is a microcytic anaemia in a patient with an inflammatory disease. The inflammatory disease will raise the serum ferritin so that a value up to 50 µg/l is suggestive of associated iron deficiency. The ethnic origin in this instance is irrelevant.[1]

(iv) e Anaemia of chronic disease. This patient with an inflammatory disease has a microcytic anaemia with an elevated serum ferritin, indicative of anaemia of chronic disease. The anaemia of chronic disease can also be associated with a normocytic normochromic anaemia.[1]

(v) b α^+ thalassaemia homozygosity. This Sudanese man has indices suggestive of thalassaemia. The low haemoglobin A_2 indicates that this is α thalassaemia not β and the degree of reduction of the MCV and MCH indicates that this is α^+ thalassaemia homozygosity not heterozygosity. The findings could also be indicative of α^0 thalassaemia heterozygosity but this is quite unlikely in this ethnic group and is not among the options offered.[2]

References

1. Bain BJ. *Blood Cells*, 5th Edn, Wiley-Blackwell, Oxford, 2015.
2. Bain BJ. *Haemoglobinopathy Diagnosis*, 2nd Edn, Blackwell Publishing, Oxford, 2006.

EMQ 9

(i) f Involved field radiotherapy with or without prior brief courses of combination chemotherapy. This patient has stage IA disease. The results of involved field radiotherapy (IFRT) are good but there is some evidence that outcome is improved by preceding this with two courses of ABVD.[1,2]

(ii) i No further treatment indicated. This patient is a young child and excision biopsy alone is an acceptable option, in order to avoid the long term risks of radiotherapy or chemotherapy.[1,2]

(iii) e Involved field radiotherapy preceded by brief courses of combination chemotherapy. This patient has stage IIB disease. Two courses of ABVD followed by IFRT is the preferred option.[1,2]

(iv) j Rituximab monotherapy. This patient is frail with extensive disease so rituximab monotherapy would be a suitable initial option.[1,2]

(v) c Combination chemotherapy plus rituximab. This patient has disease transformation and can be treated as any other patient with high grade B-cell lymphoma, with combination chemotherapy and rituximab, for example, R-CHOP.[1,2]

References

1. Fanale M (2013) Lymphocyte-predominant Hodgkin lymphoma: what is the optimal treatment? Hematology Am Soc Hematol Educ Program 2013, 2013, 406–413. PMID: 24319212.http://asheducationbook.hematologylibrary.org/content/2013/1/406.long (accessed June 2015)
2. Advani RH and Hoppe RT (2013) How I treat nodular lymphocyte predominant Hodgkin lymphoma. *Blood*, 122, 4182–4188. PMID: 24215035

EMQ 10

(i) d Dermatitis herpetiformis. This patient has dermatitis herpetiformis with the macrocytic anaemia suggesting coexisting coeliac disease. Tissue transglutaminase antibodies would be expected to be positive. A gluten-free diet is required, whether or not there is coexisting coeliac disease.[1]

(ii) g Neurofibromatosis. This young girl has features of neurofibromatosis type 1 (café-au-lait spots, freckles in unusual places (such as axillae and groins) and scoliosis), which predisposes to juvenile myelomonocytic leukaemia. Neurofibromas do not usually appear till later in childhood or during adolescence.[2]

(iii) b Blastic plasmacytoid dendritic cell neoplasm. The distinctive immunophenotype is indicative of blastic plasmacytoid dendritic cell neoplasm, which often has a cutaneous presentation.[3]

(iv) j Systemic mastocytosis. Urticaria on stroking cutaneous lesions (Darier's sign) is indicative of mastocytosis. Since the patient also has anaemia and leucopenia you can reasonably deduce that he has systemic rather than just cutaneous mastocytosis.[4]

(v) i POEMS syndrome. This patient has the POEMS (polyneuropathy organomegaly, endocrinopathy, M-protein, skin changes) syndrome.[5]

References

1. Jakes AD, Bradley S and Donlevy L (2014) Dermatitis herpetiformis. *BMJ*, 348, 34–35. PMID: 24740905
2. http://www.geneticalliance.org.uk/docs/translations/english/18-nf1-t.pdf neurofibromatosis (accessed June 2015)
3. Wrench D, Abdalla SH, Foot N and Bain BJ (2004) Teaching cases from the Royal Marsden and St Mary's Hospitals Case 28: a patient with acute leukemia with rare leukemic cells of unusual morphology. *Leuk Lymphoma*, 45, 2361–2362. PMID: 15512832
4. D'Arena G, Vita G and Musto P (2014) Darier sign and cutaneous involvement in mastocytosis. *Br J Haematol*, 167, 440. PMID: 25164313
5. Dispenzieri A (2012) POEMS syndrome: update on diagnosis, risk-stratification, and management. *Am J Hematol*, 87, 804–814. PMID: 22806697

EMQ 11

(i) i Pathogen-inactivated fresh frozen plasma plus supplementary factor VIII. There is no factor V concentrate currently available. Patients with combined factor V and factor VIII deficiency require fresh frozen plasma (FFP) and it is recommended that this be pathogen-inactivated, noting that the factor V level may be lower than in standard FFP. Because factor VIII requires a higher concentration than factor V to achieve haemostasis and because it has a shorter half- life than factor V, an additional source of factor VIII is advised, for example, recombinant factor VIII.[1]

(ii) j Tranexamic acid. Tranexamic acid is useful for excessive menstrual bleeding in patients with inherited coagulation factor deficiencies.[1]

(iii) e Either 3-product of 4-product prothrombin concentrate. Both 3-product and 4-product prothrombin concentrate can be used for factor X replacement when factor X concentrate (currently being evaluated) is not available.[1]

(iv) c Cryoprecipitate. Cryoprecipitate contains factor XIII, fibrinogen and von Willebrand factor as well as factor VIII so can be used to replace factor XIII when factor XIII concentrate is not available. A pathogen-inactivated product is preferred.

(v) d Desmopressin plus tranexamic acid. Desmopressin should be used in preference to blood derived products for minor surgery in von Willebrand disease. Tranexamic acid is a useful supplement.[1]

Reference

1. Mumford AD, Ackroyd S, Alikhan R, Bowles L, Chowdary P, Grainger J *et al*. BCSH (2014) Guideline for the diagnosis and management of the rare coagulation disorders: a United Kingdom Haemophilia Centre Doctors' Organization guideline on behalf of the British Committee for Standards in Haematology. *Br J Haematol*, 167, 304–326. PMID: 25100430

EMQ 12

(i) **f** Hairy cell leukaemia. The high forward light scatter indicates that these are fairly large cells. The immunophenotype is typical of hairy cell leukaemia.[1,2]

(ii) **b** Burkitt lymphoma. Interpretation of the immunophenotype in the light of the cytological features indicates that this is Burkitt lymphoma in leukaemic phase. Expression of CD10 is indicative of its germinal centre origin. CD38, an activation marker, is often expressed.[2]

(iii) **c** Chronic lymphocytic leukaemia. The immunophenotype is distinctive (CD5+CD23+, SmIg weak, CD79b and FMC7 negative) and is indicative of chronic lymphocytic leukaemia (CLL). CD200, a more recently introduced marker, is positive whereas it is usually negative or weak in non-Hodgkin lymphoma (it is also positive in hairy cell leukaemia). CD38 is expressed in a proportion of cases and correlates with a worse prognosis.[1,2]

(iv) **i** Plasma cell leukaemia. The immunophenotype is that of a neoplastic plasma cell. Normal plasma cells are likely to be CD19 positive and CD56 negative. Although SmIg was negative there would be light chain restricted cytoplasmic immunoglobulin. Of the markers used, CD138 is the most specific for this lineage.[2]

(v) **g** Mantle cell lymphoma. This is a CD5-positive B-cell disorder with an immunophenotype which, apart from the expression of CD5, contrasts with that of CLL.[1,2]

References

1. Leach M, Drummond M and Doig A. *Practical Flow Cytometry in Haematology Diagnosis.* Wiley-Blackwell, Chichester, 2013.
2. Bain BJ. *Leukaemia Diagnosis*, 3rd Edn, Blackwell Publishing, Oxford, 2003.

EMQ 13

(i) **d** No specific treatment.
(ii) **d** No specific treatment.
(iii) **b** Corticosteroids.
(iv) **g** platelet transfusion plus fresh frozen plasma/cryoprecipitate.
(v) **c** High dose intravenous immunoglobulin.

The management of childhood autoimmune thrombocytopenic purpura is controversial but recent opinion is that specific treatment is not indicated in most cases.[1] The advice for patient 1 is therefore that no specific treatment is indicated. However patients 3 and 5 have mucosal bleeding so are at higher risk of intracranial haemorrhage. Patient 3 can be treated with corticosteroids. However patient 5 has diabetes mellitus so it is reasonable to avoid steroids and use high dose intravenous immunoglobulin instead. Patient 2 appears to have *MYH9*-related disorder (e.g. May–Hegglin anomaly) and no treatment is indicated. Patient 4 appears to have acute promyelocytic leukaemia so requires platelet support even though the platelet count is above $10 \times 10^9/l$. He is likely to have disseminated intravascular coagulation and is likely to need management of this as well.

Reference

1. Cooper N (2014) A review of the management of childhood immune thrombocytopenia: how can we provide an evidence-based approach? *Br J Haematol*, 165, 756–767. PMID: 24761791

EMQ 14

(i) **e** Monoclonal gammopathy of undetermined significance (MGUS). The patient has MGUS. The macrocytic anaemia may be the result of early MDS, but the diagnostic criteria are not met; therefore, in addition to a diagnosis of MGUS, the designation 'idiopathic cytopenia of undetermined significance' would be appropriate.[1,2]

(ii) **c** IgM myeloma. The diagnosis is not Waldenström macroglobulinaemia but IgM myeloma. About 1% of myeloma patients have an IgM paraprotein.[3]

(iii) **b** Fanconi syndrome. Fanconi syndrome results from deposition of light chain, most often kappa, in renal tubules with resultant loss of amino acids, glucose and phosphate in the urine. Phosphate loss in turn leads to osteomalacia, accounting for the presentation with bone pain.[4]

(iv) **i** Type II cryoglobulinaemia. This patient has an IgM paraprotein with rheumatoid factor activity, complexing with polyclonal IgG.[1]

(v) **g** POEMS syndrome. The designation POEMS syndrome refers to **P**olyneuropathy, **O**rganomegaly (hepatomegaly, splenomegaly, lymphadenopathy), **E**ndocrinopathy, **M**-protein and **S**kin changes.[5]

References

1. Gertz M and Buadi FK (2012) Case vignettes and other brain teasers of monoclonal gammopathies. http://asheducationbook.hematologylibrary.org/content/2012/1/582.long (accessed June 2015)
2. Merlini G and Palladini G (2012) Differential diagnosis of monoclonal gammopathy of undetermined significance. http://asheducationbook.hematologylibrary.org/content/2012/1/595.long (accessed June 2015)
3. Ghobrial IM (2012) Are you sure this is Waldenstrom macroglobulinemia? http://asheducationbook.hematologylibrary.org/content/2012/1/586.long (accessed June 2015)
4. Fathallah-Shaykh S (2011) Fanconi syndrome. http://emedicine.medscape.com/article/981774-overview (accessed June 2015)
5. Li J and Zhou DB (2013) New advances in the diagnosis and treatment of POEMS syndrome. *Br J Haematol*, 161, 303–315. PMID: 23398538

EMQ 15

(i) g Screen partner for β thalassaemia and relevant haemoglobin-opathies. This patient has β thalassaemia heterozygosity. Her partner should be tested not only for β thalassaemia but also for relevant haemoglobinopathies, particularly haemoglobin E, haemoglobin S and haemoglobin Lepore.[1]

(ii) a No further action. Haemoglobin G-Philadelphia is of no clinical significance.

(iii) j Test patient and screen partner for α^0 thalassaemia. This patient is Chinese so may well have α^0 thalassaemia. The diagnosis should be confirmed and her partner should be screened for α^0 thalassaemia.[1]

(iv) g Screen partner for β thalassaemia and relevant haemoglobin-opathies. This patient probably has iron deficiency but her haemoglobin A_2 is at the upper end of the normal range. There is no time during pregnancy to treat with iron and repeat the test. Her partner should be screened for β thalassaemia and relevant haemoglobinopathies and unless he is haematologically normal the patient should have DNA analysis for β thalassaemia.[1]

(v) a No further action. This patient has red cell indices that are compatible with either α^0 thalassaemia heterozygosity or α^+ thalassaemia homozygosity. In this ethnic group α^0 thalassaemia is very uncommon and further testing is therefore not considered indicated. According to UK guidelines, screening and testing for α^0 thalassaemia is indicated when patients are of Chinese, Southeast Asian, Cypriot, Greek, Turkish or Sardinian ethnic origin.[2]

References

1. Bain BJ. *Haemoglobinopathy Diagnosis*, 2nd Edn, Blackwell Publishing, Oxford, 2006.
2. *Sickle Cell and Thalassaemia: Handbook for Laboratories*. http://sct.screening.nhs.uk/standardsandguidelines (accessed June 2015)

EMQ 16

(i) d Drug-induced neutropenia. The history suggests that the patient has drug-induced neutropenia due to deferiprone.[1]

(ii) h Myelodysplastic syndrome. This diagnosis is indicated by the macrocytic anaemia and the dysplastic neutrophils.[1]

(iii) a Autoimmune neutropenia. The blood film suggests large granular lymphocytic leukaemia. The frequently associated neutropenia is autoimmune in nature.[1]

(iv) b Copper deficiency. As the patient has had bariatric surgery, copper deficiency can be suspected as a cause of the neutropenia. It is important that patients who have had such surgery take the necessary vitamin supplements thereafter.[1]

(v) e Ethnic neutropenia. This mild reduction in the neutrophil count, in comparison with a Caucasian normal range, suggests ethnic neutropenia.[1]

Reference

1. Gibson C and Berliner N (2014) How we evaluate and treat neutropenia in adults. *Blood*, 124, 1251–1258. PMID: 24869938

EMQ 17

(i) c *ELANE*. This patient has severe congenital neutropenia. The majority of cases are due to a mutation in *ELANE*, the gene encoding neutrophil elastase.[1]

(ii) a *DARC*. This patient has ethnic neutropenia. This has been linked to abnormalities in Duffy antigens and mutations in *DARC*.[2]

(iii) h *RPS19*. This patient has Diamond–Blackfan anaemia. The gene most commonly implicated is *RPS19*, mutation of which is responsible for about a quarter of cases.[3]

(iv) c *ELANE*. This patient has cyclical neutropenia. Like the majority of cases of severe congenital neutropenia, this is due to mutation in *ELANE* and occasionally the two conditions occur in the same family.[1]

(v) f *MYH9*. This patient has the May–Hegglin anomaly and, in addition, chronic kidney disease and deafness, known as Epstein syndrome, part of the spectrum of *MYH9*-related disorders.[4]

With the exception of *MYH11*, all the other genes listed have been implicated in inherited haematological disorders.

References

1. Newburger PE, Pindyck TN, Zhu Z, Bolyard AA, Aprikyan AA, Dale DC *et al.* (2010) Cyclic neutropenia and severe congenital neutropenia in patients with a shared ELANE mutation and paternal haplotype: evidence for phenotype determination by modifying genes. *Pediatr Blood Cancer*, 55, 314–317. PMID: 20582973

2. Grann VR, Ziv E, Joseph CK, Neugut AI, Wei Y, Jacobson JS *et al.* (2008) Duffy (Fy), DARC, and neutropenia among women from the United States, Europe and the Caribbean. *Br J Haematol*, 143, 288–293. PMID: 18710383

3. Gazda HT and Sieff CA (2006) Recent insights into the pathogenesis of Diamond–Blackfan anaemia. *Br J Haematol*, 135, 149–157. PMID: 16942586

4. Balduini CL, Pecci A and Savoia A (2011) Recent advances in the understanding and management of MYH9-related inherited thrombocytopenias. *Br J Haematol*, 154, 161–174. PMID: 21542825

EMQ 18

(i) **f** Folic acid deficiency. The patient's history suggests coeliac disease. Vitamin B_{12} deficiency is a possible cause of megaloblastic anaemia in coeliac disease but folic acid deficiency is more common so is the preferred answer.[1]

(ii) **j** Vitamin B_{12} deficiency. Apart from the vitamin B_{12} within the normal range, all the features of this patient point to pernicious anaemia. It is important to be aware that not all patients with pernicious anaemia have a low serum B_{12} and that some assays give falsely elevated results in the presence of intrinsic factor antibodies.[2]

(iii) **a** 5q– syndrome. The combination of macrocytosis, thrombocytosis and hypolobated megakaryocytes points to the 5q– syndrome.[3]

(iv) **b** Autoimmune haemolytic anaemia. The clinical presentation suggests that the anaemia is due to autoimmune haemolytic anaemia occurring as a complication of chronic lymphocytic leukaemia. The macrocytosis reflects reticulocytosis.

(v) **h** Refractory cytopenia with multilineage dysplasia. This patient with a myelodysplastic syndrome has dysplasia in two lineages (erythroid and granulocytic) and the diagnosis is therefore refractory cytopenia with multilineage dysplasia rather than refractory anaemia with ring sideroblasts.[4] In the 2008 WHO classification this category includes cases with and without 15% or more ring sideroblasts.

References

1. Halfdanarson TR, Litzow MR and Murray JA (2007) Hematologic manifestations of celiac disease. *Blood*, 109, 412–421. PMID: 16973955
2. Carmel R and Agrawal YP (2012) Failures of cobalamin assays in pernicious anemia. *N Engl J Med*, 367, 385–386. PMID: 22830482
3. Jädersten M (2010) Pathophysiology and treatment of the myelodysplastic syndrome with isolated 5q deletion. *Haematologica*, 95, 348–351. PMID: 20207839
4. Brunning RD, Bennett JM, Matutes E, Orazi A, Vardiman JW and Thiele J. Refractory cytopenia with multilineage dysplasia. *In* Swerdlow SH, Campo E, Harris NL, Jaffe ES, Pileri SA, Stein H, Thiele J and Vardiman JW (Eds) *World Health Organization Classification of Tumours of Haematopoietic and Lymphoid Tissues*. IARC Press, Lyon, 2008, pp 98–99.

EMQ 19

(i) e Mycosis fungoides. The clinical and histological feature without circulating neoplastic cells indicate that this is mycosis fungoides not Sézary syndrome.[1]

(ii) i Sézary syndrome. With more than 5% circulating Sézary cells, the patient meets the criteria for this diagnosis. Pautrier's microabscesses are shown on skin biopsy.[1]

(iii) f Myeloid sarcoma. This patient has blast transformation of chronic myelogenous leukaemia, manifesting as an isolated myeloid sarcoma.

(iv) j T-prolymphocytic leukaemia. Skin infiltration is present in about a fifth of patients with T-prolymphocytic leukaemia (T-PLL). Pleural effusions are less common. Expression of CD7 helps to distinguish T-PLL from other T-cell lymphomas. About a quarter of patients show co-expression of CD4 and CD8.[2]

(v) a Adult T-cell leukaemia/lymphoma. The clinical, haematological and histological features point to a diagnosis of adult T-cell leukaemia/lymphoma (ATLL). Note that Pautrier's microabscesses are not specific for Sézary syndrome. They are also quite common in ATLL[3] and the other features are much more suggestive of ATLL.

References

1. Hwang ST, Janik JE, Jaffe ES and Wilson WH (2008) Mycosis fungoides and Sézary syndrome. *Lancet*, 371, 945–957. PMID: 18342689
2. Matutes E, Brito-Babapulle V, Swansbury J, Ellis J, Morilla R, Dearden C et al. (1991) Clinical and laboratory features of 78 cases of T-prolymphocytic leukemia. *Blood*, 78, 3269–3274. PMID: 1742486
3. Ohshima K, Jaffe ES and Kikuchi M. Adult T-cell leukaemia/lymphoma. *In* Swerdlow SH, Campo E, Harris NL, Jaffe ES, Pileri SA, Stein H, Thiele J and Vardiman JW (Eds) *World Health Organization Classification of Tumours of Haematopoietic and Lymphoid Tissues*, IARC Press, Lyon, 2008, pp 281–284.

EMQ 20

(i) i Haemoglobin H disease. This is a typical example of this condition.[1]

(ii) a α^0 thalassaemia heterozygosity. The haematological abnormality is too marked to be α^+ thalassaemia heterozygosity and is indicative of α^0 thalassaemia heterozygosity. Another possibility would be α^+ thalassaemia homozygosity but this is not among the options available. One cannot exclude εγδβ thalassaemia heterozygosity but this is quite rare so is not the most likely diagnosis.[1]

(iii) j Hereditary persistence of fetal haemoglobin. This patient has a normal blood count but an increased haemoglobin F and a reduced haemoglobin A_2. Since the indices are normal, the diagnosis must be hereditary persistence of fetal haemoglobin (HPFH) rather than δβ thalassaemia heterozygosity. This an example of the Afro-American type of HPFH, HPFH-1.[1]

(iv) h Haemoglobin E heterozygosity. The thalassaemic indices are typical of haemoglobin E trait. It is important to realise that haemoglobin A_2 is never as high as this and there must be a variant haemoglobin present with the same retention time as haemoglobin A_2. The 28% represents the haemoglobin E plus haemoglobin A_2. Haemoglobin E is present as a relatively low percentage (considering that it is a β chain variant) because the β^E chain is synthesised at a reduced rate.[1]

(v) c β thalassaemia heterozygosity. This is a totally typical example of β thalassaemia trait.[1]

Reference

1. Bain BJ, Wild BJ, Stephens AD and Phelan LA. *Variant Haemoglobins: a Guide to Identification.* Wiley-Blackwell, Oxford. 2010.

EMQ 21

(i) g Fanconi anaemia. Fanconi anaemia can result from mutation in at least 16 genes.[1] Thumb abnormalities and café-au-lait spots are common.

(ii) d Diamond–Blackfan anaemia. Pure red cell aplasia with increased haemoglobin F and adenosine deaminase are typical of this condition.[2] Somatic abnormalities are sometimes present.

(iii) i Shwachman–Diamond syndrome. This disorder is characterised by a fatty pancreas with steatorrhoea and neutropenia.[2] Anaemia and thrombocytopenia are less common.

(iv) j Thrombocytopenia with absent radii. In this condition the platelet count generally improves after the first year of life and may reach normal or near normal levels.[3]

(v) e Dyskeratosis congenita. The most common genetic defect underlying this condition is mutation in *DKC1*, which causes X-linked disease.[4]

References

1. Longerich S, Li J, Xiong Y, Sung P and Kupfer GM (2014) Stress and DNA repair biology of the Fanconi anemia pathway. *Blood*, 124, 2812–2819 PMID: 25237197
2. Ruggero D and Shimamura A (2014) Marrow failure: a window into ribosome biology. *Blood*, 124, 2784–2792. PMID: 25237201
3. De Ybarrondo and Barratt MS (2011) Thrombocytopenia absent radius syndrome. *Pediatr Rev*, 32, 399–400. PMID: 21885665
4. Townsley DM, Dumitriu B and Young NS (2014) Bone marrow failure and the telomeropathies. *Blood*, 124, 2775–2783. PMID: 25237198

EMQ 22

(i) **e** Acaeruloplasminaemia. The associated features identify this as acaeruloplasminaemia. Caeruloplasmin is essential for oxidising Fe^{++} to Fe^{+++} and for export of iron from cells. Deficiency leads to iron overload.[1]

(ii) **h** Hypotransferrinaemia. This patient has iron deficient erythropoiesis as a result of hypotransferrinaemia. An increase of non-transferrin bound iron leads to early iron overload.[2–4]

(iii) **d** $\delta\beta$ thalassaemia. This patient has hypochromia and microcytosis so the diagnosis is $\delta\beta$ thalassaemia not hereditary persistence of fetal haemoglobin.[5]

(iv) **f** Congenital sideroblastic anaemia. This case is based on the patient described by Aguiar *et al.* (2014).[6] The dimorphic film and iron overload in the mother indicate an X-linked sideroblastic anaemia in the child; an *ALAS2* mutation is likely. Dimorphism may be more marked in female heterozygotes in comparison with male hemizygotes, Skewed inactivation of X chromosomes can lead to sideroblastic anaemia and iron overload in females.

(v) **a** α^0 thalassaemia heterozygosity. This patient has α^0 thalassaemia heterozygosity. The reduction in the MCH is too severe to be attributable to α^+ thalassaemia heterozygosity and β thalassaemia heterozygosity has been excluded. α^+ thalassaemia homozygosity is not excluded but is not an option offered.[5]

References

1. Harris ZL, Takahashi Y, Miyajima H, Serizawa M, MacGillivray RTA and Gitlin JD (1995) Aceruloplasminemia: molecular characterization of this disorder of iron metabolism. *Proc Nat Acad Sci USA*, 92, 2549–2543.
2. Donker AE, Raymakers RA, Vlasveld LT, van Barneveld T, Terink R, Dors N *et al.* (2014) Practice guidelines for the diagnosis and management of microcytic anemias due to genetic disorders of iron metabolism or heme synthesis. *Blood*, 123, 3873–3886. PMID: 24665134
3. Iolascon A, De Falco L and Beaumont C (2009) Molecular basis of inherited microcytic anemia due to defects in iron acquisition or heme synthesis. *Haematologica*, 94, 395–408. PMID: 19181781
4. Camaschella C (2013) How I manage patients with atypical microcytic anaemia. *Br J Haematol*, 160, 12–24. PMID: 23057559
5. Bain BJ. *Haemoglobinopathy Diagnosis*, 2nd Edn, Blackwell Publishing, Oxford, 2006.
6. Aguiar E, Freitas MI and Barbot J (2014) Different haematological picture of congenital sideroblastic anaemia in a hemizygote and a heterozygote. *Br J Haematol*, 166, 469. PMID: 24862439

EMQ 23

(i) b Drug withdrawal. This patient has gemcitabine-induced microangiopathy. Drug withdrawal is indicated but rituximab is not known to be of benefit.[1,2]

(ii) d Eculizumab. This patient has complement factor H deficiency, which can be managed with eculizumab. Vaccination against meningococcus should be carried out.[1,2]

(iii) g Haemodialysis. This child has haemolytic uraemic syndrome and requires haemodialysis.[1,2]

(iv) h Plasma exchange plus corticosteroids. This patient has thrombotic thrombocytopenic purpura. Plasma exchange is indicated rather than plasma infusion and is usually supplemented with corticosteroids. If necessary, plasma infusion can be used initially while plasma exchange is being arranged. Treatment should not be delayed while waiting for the results of the ADAMTS13 assay.[1,2]

(v) e Eculizumab, followed by immunosuppression. This patient has complement-mediated microangiopathy as a result of an acquired, antibody-mediated deficiency of factor H. Because of the high costs of eculizumab, it is reasonable to follow this initial therapy with immunosuppression to reduce the antibody titre.[1,2]

References

1. George JN and Nester CM (2014) Syndromes of thrombotic microangiopathy. *N Engl J Med*, 371, 654–666. PMID: 25119611
2. Scully M, Hunt BJ, Benjamin S, Liesner R, Rose P, Peyvandi F *et al*. British Committee for Standards in Haematology (2012) Guidelines on the diagnosis and management of thrombotic thrombocytopenic purpura and other thrombotic microangiopathies. *Br J Haematol*, 158, 323–335. PMID: 22624596

EMQ 24

(i) **i** t(12;21)(p13;q22). This child has B-lineage lymphoblastic leukaemia/lymphoma. In this age range the two most common cytogenetic abnormalities are high hyperdiploidy and a cryptic t(12;21)(p13;q22). The latter is therefore the correct answer. CD13 is not infrequently expressed.[1,2]

(ii) **e** t(8;14)(q24;q32).This patient has Burkitt lymphoma and the most frequently observed translocation is t(8;14)(q24;q32).[1,2]

(iii) **j** t(14;18)(q32;q21). This patient has follicular lymphoma and the most frequently observed translocation is t(14;18) (q32;q21).[1,2]

(iv) **h** t(11;14)(q13;q32). This patient has mantle cell lymphoma and the most frequently observed translocation is t(11;14) (q13;q32).[1,2]

(v) **f** t(9;22)(q34;q11.2). This patient has B-lineage lymphoblastic leukaemia/lymphoma. In this age range, t(9;22)(q34;q11.2) is by far the most common translocation and the immunophenotype, including the expression of CD25, is typical of Ph-positive acute lymphoblastic leukaemia.[1,2] Aberrant expression of CD13 and CD33 is common.

References

1. Swerdlow SH, Campo E, Harris NL, Jaffe ES, Pileri SA, Stein H, Thiele J and Vardiman JW. *World Health Organization Classification of Tumours of Haematopoietic and Lymphoid Tissues*, 4th Edn, IARC Press, Lyon, 2008.
2. Matutes E, Bain BJ and Wotherspoon A. *An Atlas of Investigation and Diagnosis: Lymphoid Malignancies*. Clinical Publishing, Oxford, 2007.

EMQ 25

(i) d Eosinophilic granulomatosis with polyangiitis. This patient has eosinophilic granulomatosis with polyangiitis, previously known as the Churg–Strauss syndrome.[1] Patients with eosinophilia may be referred to a haematologist so an awareness of non-haematological causes of eosinophilia is necessary.

(ii) e Hodgkin lymphoma. The presence of unilateral hilar lymphadenopathy and alcohol-related symptoms suggests a reactive eosinophilia due to underlying Hodgkin lymphoma.

(iii) a Allergic bronchopulmonary aspergillosis. The clinical history and the radiological findings suggest this diagnosis rather than an aspergilloma.[2]

(iv) i Parasitic infection. The clinical and haematological features suggest schistosomiasis (specifically *Schistosoma haematobium* infection).

(v) g Myeloid neoplasm with rearrangement of *PDGFRA*. The deletion of the *CHIC2* gene shows that this case of chronic eosinophilic leukaemia is due to a *FIP1L1-PDGFRA* fusion gene, the fusion gene being formed as a result of an interstitial deletion that includes *CHIC2*.[3] The presence of increased mast cells should not lead to a mistaken diagnosis of systemic mastocytosis.

References

1. Mahr A, Moosig F, Neumann T, Szczeklik W, Taillé C, Vaglio A and Zwerina J (2014) Eosinophilic granulomatosis with polyangiitis (Churg-Strauss): evolutions in classification, etiopathogenesis, assessment and management. *Curr Opin Rheumatol*, 26, 16–23. PMID: 24257370

2. Harman EM (2014) Aspergillosis. http://emedicine.medscape.com/article/296052-overview (accessed June 2015)

3. Bain BJ, Gilliland DG, Horny H-P and Vardiman JW. Myeloid and lymphoid neoplasms with eosinophilia and abnormalities of PDGFRA, PDGFRB and FGFR1. *In* Swerdlow SH, Campo E, Harris NL, Jaffe ES, Pileri SA, Stein H, Thiele J and Vardiman JW (Eds) *World Health Organization Classification of Tumours of Haematopoietic and Lymphoid Tissues*, 4th Edn, IARC Press, Lyon, 2008, pp 68–73.

EMQ 26

(i) **g** Paroxysmal cold haemoglobinuria. The blood film is typical of PCH[1] and, although the haemolysis is IgG mediated, often a DAT detects only complement. The reticulocyte count is often not increased early after onset.

(ii) **b** Delayed haemolytic transfusion reaction. This patient has recently had major surgery so it is highly likely that he was transfused. The mixed field agglutination indicates a delayed transfusion reaction.

(iii) **i** Unstable haemoglobin. A low MCHC and a low platelet count are sometimes seen in patients with an unstable haemoglobin, the low MCHC being attributed to removal of Heinz bodies by the spleen. G6PD deficiency is unlikely in a female (except in high prevalence areas) and the splenomegaly and elevated bilirubin and LDH in the interval between episodes of overt haemolysis would not be expected.

(iv) **a** Chronic cold haemagglutinin disease. The history is compatible with cold-induced haemolysis and it is highly likely that the elevated MCV is factitious, as a result of a cold agglutinin. Megaloblastic anaemia is improbable, given the history.

(v) **c** Epstein–Barr virus-related cold antibody-mediated haemolysis. This patient has infectious mononucleosis. The associated haemolysis is due to a cold antibody, which in this condition often, but not always,[2] has anti-i specificity.

References

1. Bharadwaj V, Chakravorty S and Bain BJ (2011) The cause of sudden anemia revealed by the blood film. *Am J Hematol*, 87, 520. PMID: 21953885
2. Wilkinson LS, Petz LD and Garratty G (1973) Reappraisal of the role of anti-i in haemolytic anaemia in infectious mononucleosis. *Br J Haematol*, 25, 715–722. PMID: 4128232

EMQ 27

(i) a Chronic renal failure. Renal failure should be suspected in a patient of this age with sickle cell disease who presents with the slow fall of Hb.

(ii) g Normal for this patient. This Hb is within the expected range for someone with sickle cell anaemia. There is no reason to think that it relates to the recent infection.

(iii) j Splenic sequestration. This is not hypersplenism but more specifically splenic sequestration, a complication of sickle cell disease that is seen in young children before recurrent infarction has led to fibrosis of the spleen.

(iv) h Parvovirus B19 infection. The very low reticulocyte count makes parvovirus B19 infection likely. Early erythroid precursors are infected by the virus and there is an arrest of erythropoiesis.

(v) d Hyperhaemolysis. The Hb is significantly below the pretransfusion level. This makes a simple delayed haemolytic transfusion reaction an inadequate explanation and indicates that haemolysis of the patient's own erythrocytes has occurred. The mechanisms of hyperhaemolysis are not clear.[1] The phenomenon has been described in patients with and without sickle cell disease, and in those with and without detectable alloantibodies.

Reference

1. Win N, New H, Lee E and de la Fuente J (2008) Hyperhemolysis syndrome in sickle cell disease: Case report (recurrent episode) and literature review. *Transfusion*, 48, 1231–1238. PMID: 18373500

EMQ 28

(i) **c** t(1;22)(p13;q13). This is a typical case of childhood acute megakaryoblastic leukaemia associated with t(1;22). The bone marrow blast count is often relatively low and there may be bone marrow fibrosis.[1]

(ii) **d** t(5;12)(q31-33;p12). This patient has chronic myelomonocytic leukaemia with eosinophilia, consistent with *PDGFRB* rearrangement associated with t(5;12). The presence of monocytosis and the absence of basophilia make chronic myelogeneous leukaemia with t(9;22) unlikely.[2]

(iii) **e** t(6;9)(p23;q34). This patient has acute myelomonocytic leukaemia with basophilic as well as neutrophilic differentiation and trilineage dysplasia, all features that may be seen in association with t(6;9).[1]

(iv) **j** t(15;17)(q22;q12). This patient has epistaxis and bruising despite the platelet count being 30×10^9/l. This suggests either defective platelet function or a coagulation abnormality; in this case it indicates disseminated intravascular coagulation associated with the variant form of acute promyelocytic leukaemia. Note that the Hb is sometimes normal or near normal in this type of leukaemia.[1]

(v) **b** inv(16)(p13.1q22). This patient has the cytological features expected with inv(16)(p13.1q22) or t(16;16)(p13.1;q22).[1] Note in passing that in cytogenetic notation there is a semicolon separating the breakpoints in a translocation but not in an inversion.

References

1. Arber DA, Brunning RD, Le Beau MM, Falini B, Vardiman JW, Porwit A, Thiele J and Bloomfield CD. Acute myeloid leukaemia with recurrent genetic abnormalities. *In* Swerdlow SH, Campo E, Harris NL, Jaffe ES, Pileri SA, Stein H, Thiele J and Vardiman JW (Eds) *World Health Organization Classification of Tumours of Haematopoietic and Lymphoid Tissues*, 4th Edn, IARC Press, Lyon, 2008, pp 110–123.
2. Bain BJ, Gilliland DG, Horny H-P and Vardiman JW. Myeloid and lymphoid neoplasms with eosinophilia and abnormalities of PDGFRA, PDGFRB and FGFR1. *In* Swerdlow SH, Campo E, Harris NL, Jaffe ES, Pileri SA, Stein H, Thiele J and Vardiman JW (Eds) *World Health Organization Classification of Tumours of Haematopoietic and Lymphoid Tissues*, 4th Edn, IARC Press, Lyon, 2008, pp 68–73.

EMQ 29

(i) g Haemolysis due to invasion and rosetting of erythrocytes. In falciparum malaria haemolysis is attributable not only to parasite invasion of red cells followed by lysis but also to rosetting of infected with non-infected red cells mediated by ABO antigens and with resultant complement fixation and accelerated clearance of non-parasitised as well as parasitised erythrocytes.[1]

(ii) a Arrest of erythropoiesis. This patient has parvovirus B19 infection leading to arrest of erythropoiesis at the proerythroblast stage of maturation.[2] Entry to the red cell precursors is through the P antigen. Because of the shortened red cell life span in hereditary spherocytosis, anaemia develops before the immune response that clears the virus has had time to develop.

(iii) i Microangiopathic haemolytic anaemia. The history suggests haemolytic uraemic syndrome due to infection by *Escherichia coli* O157:H7. Endothelial damage leads to microangiopathic haemolytic anaemia and acute kidney injury.

(iv) b Erythrocyte membrane damage by exotoxin. The history suggests *Clostridium perfringens* septicaemia. The red cell membrane is damage by a bacterial exotoxin that has lecithinase activity.[1]

(v) d Haemolysis due to a cold agglutinin with anti-I specificity. The clinicopathological features suggest *Mycoplasma pneumoniae* infection. The cold agglutinin that causes haemolysis usually has anti-I specificity.[1]

References
1. McCullough J (2014) RBCs as targets of infection. *Hematology*, 2014, 404–409.
2. Young NS and Brown KE (2004) Parvovirus B19. *N Engl J Med*, 350, 586–597. PMID: 14762186

EMQ 30

(i) g Phytosterolaemia. Also known as sitosterolaemia, this is an autosomal recessive condition in which there is increased absorption of cholesterol and plant sterols. The overhydrated and dehydrated variants of stomatocytosis are not associated with large platelets.[1]

(ii) e Hereditary pyropoikilocytosis. It is likely that her mother has the low expression allele of the alpha spectrin gene, α spectrin[LELY]. It should be noted that reduced binding of eosin-5-maleimide is not specific for hereditary spherocytosis, being found also in hereditary pyropoikilocytosis and South-east Asian ovalocytosis.[2]

(iii) f Overhydrated hereditary stomatocytosis. Splenectomy is contraindicated in this condition because of the thrombotic complications that often follow.[3] Dehydrated hereditary stomatocytosis often does not show numerous stomatocytes

(iv) h Pyrimidine 5' nucleotidase deficiency. Prominent basophilic stippling is typical.

(v) c Glucose-6-phosphate dehydrogenase (G6PD) deficiency. This diagnosis is much more likely than heterozygosity for an unstable haemoglobin, such as haemoglobin Köln.

References

1. Rees DC, Iolascon A, Carella M, O'Marcaigh AS Kendra JR, Jowitt SN et al. (2005) Stomatocytic haemolysis and macrothrombocytopenia (Mediterranean stomatocytosis/macrothrombocytopenia) is the haematological presentation of phytosterolaemia. *Br J Haematol*, 130, 297–309. PMID: 16029460
2. King MJ, Telfer P, MacKinnon H, Langabeer L, McMahon C, Darbyshire P and Dhermy D (2008) Using the eosin-5-maleimide binding test in the differential diagnosis of hereditary spherocytosis and hereditary pyropoikilocytosis. *Cytometry B Clin Cytom*, 74, 244–250. PMID: 18454487
3. Delaunay J (2007) The molecular basis of hereditary red cell membrane disorders. *Blood Rev*, 21, 1–20. PMID: 16730867
4. Rees DC, Duley DA and Marinaki AM (2003) Pyrimidine 5' nucleotidase deficiency. *Br J Haematol*, 120, 375–383. PMID: 12580951

Index

Topics are indexed by section (SBA, EMQ) and question number. Readers should refer to the relevant section under each topic. For SBA questions, questions 1–31 are particularly suitable for MRCP part 1, questions 32–50 are particularly suitable for MRCP part 2, and questions 51–120 for haematology specialist trainees. SBAs 19, 23, 52, 55, 63, 79, 81, 86, 87, 88, 96, 101, 104, 105 and 108 are particular suitable for paediatric trainees. Many of the EMQs have a paediatric component, but EMQs 13 and 21 are of particular relevance.

abdominal pain SBA 19
ABVD regimen EMQ 6
acaeruloplasminaemia EMQ 22
acrocyanosis SBA 68, EMQ 26
activated partial thromboplastin time (APTT) SBA 12, SBA 21, SBA 25, SBA 27, SBA 49, SBA 55
activated prothrombin complex SBA 72
acute haemolytic transfusion reaction EMQ 3
acute lymphoblastic leukaemia SBA 14, SBA 81
acute myeloid leukaemia SBA 13, SBA 31, SBA 83
acute myelomonocytic leukaemia EMQ 28
acute promyelocytic leukaemia SBA 77
ADAMTS13 SBA 73

ADAMTS13 antibody SBA 9, SBA 80
adult T-cell leukaemia/lymphoma SBA 1, SBA 51, SBA 65, EMQ 1, EMQ 19
alanine transaminase SBA 29
ALAS2 mutation SBA 89
alcoholic cirrhosis SBA 50
alemtuzumab SBA 62, SBA 113
allergic bronchopulmonary aspergillosis EMQ 25
alloimmune thrombocytopenia EMQ 5
allopurinol SBA 41, SBA 79
alopecia SBA 51
α^+ thalassaemia homozygosity EMQ 8
α^0 thalassaemia SBA 98, EMQ 15
  heterozygosity EMQ 20, EMQ 22

anaemia SBA 18
  aplastic SBA 62
  autoimmune haemolytic
    EMQ 18
  of chronic disease SBA 5,
    SBA 30, SBA 91, EMQ 8
  congenital sideroblastic
    EMQ 22
  Fanconi EMQ 21
  iron deficiency SBA 5, SBA 8,
    SBA 11, SBA 88, EMQ 8
  megaloblastic SBA 16, SBA 18,
    SBA 22
  microangiopathic haemolytic
    SBA 73, EMQ 29
  pernicious SBA 100
  warm autoimmune haemolytic
    SBA 113
anaphylactic transfusion reaction
    EMQ 3
angioimmunoblastic T-cell
    lymphoma EMQ 1
anisocytosis SBA 6, SBA 22,
    SBA 23, SBA 108
anorexia nervosa SBA 4
anti-thrombin activity
    SBA 93
antibodies
  ADAMTS13 SBA 9, SBA 80
  IgA anti-tissue transflutaminase
    SBA 8
  intrinsic factor SBA 32, SBA
    100
antiphospholipid syndrome SBA
    44
antiretroviral therapy EMQ 6
aphasia SBA 47
aplastic anaemia SBA 62
argatroban SBA 107

aspergillosis, allergic bronchopul-
    monary EMQ 25
aspirin SBA 82, SBA 103,
    SBA 112
atrial fibrillation SBA 47, SBA 93
atypical haemolytic uraemic
    syndrome SBA 36, SBA 73
Auer rods SBA 31
autoimmune haemolytic anaemia
    EMQ 18
  warm SBA 113
autoimmune lymphoproliferative
    syndrome SBA 63
autoimmune neutropenia
    EMQ 16
autoimmune thrombocytopenic
    purpura SBA 18, SBA 86
Ayurvedic medicine SBA 6

B-cell lymphoma SBA 92
  unclassifiable SBA 67
B-lineage lymphoblastic leukae-
    mia/lymphoma EMQ 24
bariatric surgery SBA 94
basophilic stippling SBA 6
BCR-ABL1 SBA 58, SBA 75,
    SBA 116
BEACOPP regimen EMQ 6
Bernard-Soulier syndrome
    EMQ 5
β thalassaemia SBA 23, SBA 118,
    EMQ 15
  heterozygosity SBA 99, EMQ 8,
    EMQ 20
β⁺ thalassaemia SBA 95
β⁰ thalassaemia SBA 108
bilirubin SBA 29, SBA 35
biochemistry SBA 79
blast cells SBA 31

blastic plasmacytoid dendritic cell
 neoplasm SBA 64, EMQ 10
bleomycin SBA 14, SBA 40,
 EMQ 6
blood transfusion SBA 3, SBA 57,
 SBA 59
 reactions *see* transfusion
 reactions
blurred vision SBA 16
bone marrow
 aspirate SBA 6
 hypocellularity SBA 4
bone pain SBA 114
Borrelia burgdorferi EMQ 7
brain tumour SBA 92
breast cancer SBA 14, SBA 34,
 SBA 71, SBA 85, SBA 116
bruising SBA 86, EMQ 13,
 EMQ 28
Bruton's tyrosine kinase inhibitors
 SBA 76
Burkitt lymphoma SBA 41,
 SBA 79, SBA 85, EMQ 12,
 EMQ 24
busulphan SBA 90

C3 SBA 56
café-au-lait spots EMQ 21
calcium SBA 33
CALR mutation SBA 58
cancer *see* neoplasms
carpal tunnel syndrome SBA 94
CD1a SBA 87
CD34 SBA 70
CD64 SBA 77
CHAD$_2$DS$_2$-VASc score SBA 46
Charcot-Leyden crystals EMQ 28
Chlamydophila psittaci SBA 69,
 EMQ 7

cholecystectomy SBA 59
cholesterol embolisation SBA 39
chronic eosinophilic leukaemia
 SBA 75
chronic lymphocytic leukaemia
 SBA 1, SBA 76, SBA 110,
 EMQ 12
chronic myelogenous leukaemia
 SBA 52, SBA 116
chronic myelomonocytic
 leukaemia EMQ 28
ciclosporin SBA 62
Clostridium perfringens SBA 83,
 EMQ 29
coeliac disease SBA 8, SBA 15
cold antibody-mediated
 haemolysis EMQ 26
cold haemagglutinin disease
 SBA 68
 chronic EMQ 26
colestyramine SBA 25
combination chemotherapy
 SBA 53, SBA 117, EMQ 9
computed tomography (CT)
 SBA 44
congenital heart disease
 SBA 105
congenital sideroblastic anaemia
 EMQ 22
copper deficiency SBA 94,
 EMQ 16
coronary artery disease SBA 14
corticosteroids SBA 72, SBA 86,
 EMQ 13, EMQ 23
cough SBA 28
CREST SBA 11
cryoglobulinaemia, type II
 EMQ 14
cryoprecipitate EMQ 11, EMQ 13

cyclophosphamide SBA 37,
SBA 40, SBA 72, SBA 110,
EMQ 6
cytopenia, refractory with multilineage dysplasia EMQ 18
D dimer SBA 12, SBA 27, SBA 38
dabigatran SBA 84, SBA 93
dacarbazine SBA 14, EMQ 6
danazol SBA 97
dapsone SBA 106
DARC EMQ 17
Darier's sign EMQ 10
deep vein thrombosis SBA 7,
SBA 21, SBA 38, SBA 107,
SBA 109
defibrotide SBA 90
delayed haemolytic transfusion
reaction EMQ 3
δβ-thalassaemia SBA 108,
EMQ 22
dengue fever SBA 27
dermatitis herpetiformis SBA
106, EMQ 10
desferasirox SBA 78
desmopressin SBA 74, EMQ 11
diabetes insipidus SBA 87
diabetes mellitus SBA 24
Diamond-Blackfan syndrome
EMQ 21
diffuse large B-cell lymphoma
SBA 37
direct antiglobulin test SBA 56,
SBA 63, SBA 105
DNA antibodies SBA 18
Döhle bodies SBA 119
double negative lymphocytes
SBA 63
double vision SBA 42

Down syndrome SBA 81,
SBA 104
doxorubicin SBA 14, SBA 37,
SBA 40, EMQ 6
doxycycline SBA 69
drug-induced neutropenia
EMQ 16
dyserythropoiesis SBA 6, SBA 70
dyskeratosis congenita EMQ 21
dysphasia SBA 46
eculizumab SBA 56, SBA 73,
EMQ 23
efalizumab SBA 2
ELANE EMQ 17
eosinophilia SBA 28, SBA 45
eosinophilic granulomatosis with
polyangiitis EMQ 25
epistaxis EMQ 28
Epstein-Barr virus EMQ 7,
EMQ 26
erythrocyte sedimentation
rate (ESR) SBA 1, SBA 5,
SBA 20, SBA 42, SBA 53,
EMQ 6, EMQ 25
erythroderma SBA 51
erythropoietin SBA 54, SBA 97,
SBA 103
Escherichia coli O104:H4
SBA 9
Escherichia coli O157:H7
SBA 9
ethnic neutropenia EMQ 16
etoposide EMQ 6
exchange transfusion SBA 101
extranodal marginal zone
lymphoma SBA 69
extranodal NK/T-cell lymphoma,
nasal type EMQ 1

factor VIIa, recombinant SBA 72,
   EMQ 2
factor VIII EMQ 11
factor VIII inhibitor SBA 72
factor XI concentrate EMQ 2
factor XI deficiency SBA 49
Fanconi anaemia EMQ 21
Fanconi syndrome EMQ 14
fatigue SBA 100, SBA 120,
   EMQ 28
felodipine SBA 47
ferritin SBA 5, SBA 23, SBA 30,
   SBA 78, SBA 89
fetal haemoglobin *see*
   haemoglobin F
fibrinogen SBA 25
   concentrate EMQ 2
fludarabine SBA 110
fluid restriction SBA 40
fluid therapy SBA 41
folate
   deficiency SBA 16, EMQ 18
   serum SBA 8
   supplements SBA 15
follicular lymphoma EMQ 24
fresh frozen plasma
   pathogen-inactivated EMQ 11
   solvent detergent-treated
      SBA 80, EMQ 2

gelofusine SBA 80
gemcitabine-induced
   microangiopathy EMQ 23
giant cell arteritis SBA 20
glucose-6-phosphate
   dehydrogenase deficiency
   SBA 17, SBA 79, SBA 106,
   EMQ 30
graft-versus-host disease SBA 13

HAART therapy SBA 117
haematocrit SBA 5, SBA 6,
   SBA 11
haematuria SBA 19, EMQ 25
haemodialysis EMQ 23
haemoglobin
   transfusion threshold SBA 3
   unstable EMQ 26
haemoglobin A_{1c} SBA 24
haemoglobin A_2 SBA 96, SBA 98,
   SBA 99, SBA 108
haemoglobin C disease
   EMQ 27
haemoglobin D-Punjab trait
   SBA 111
haemoglobin E SBA 98
   heterozygosity EMQ 20
haemoglobin F SBA 61, SBA 96,
   SBA 108
   hereditary persistence
      EMQ 20
haemoglobin G-Philadelphia
   SBA 111, EMQ 15
haemoglobin H disease SBA 23,
   EMQ 20
haemoglobin O-Arab SBA 118
haemoglobin S SBA 111,
   SBA 118
haemoglobin S/β^+ thalassaemia
   compound heterozygosity
   SBA 95
haemoglobinuria
   paroxysmal cold EMQ 26
   paroxysmal nocturnal SBA 56
haemolytic anaemia
   autoimmune EMQ 18
   microangiopathic SBA 73,
      EMQ 29
   warm autoimmune SBA 113

haemolytic disease of newborn
SBA 101
haemolytic transfusion reaction
acute EMQ 3
delayed EMQ 26
haemolytic uraemic syndrome
SBA 9, EMQ 4, EMQ 23,
EMQ 29
atypical SBA 36, SBA 73
haemophilia SBA 72
haemopoietic stem cell transplant
SBA 13, SBA 96
haemoptysis SBA 11
hairy cell leukaemia EMQ 12
Hashimoto thyroiditis SBA 32
headache SBA 28, SBA 29,
SBA 42
Heinz bodies SBA 17
Helicobacter heilmanii EMQ 7
hemiparesis SBA 47
Henoch-Schönlein purpura
SBA 19
heparin, low molecular weight
SBA 82
heparin-induced
thrombocytopenia SBA 107
hepatitis B SBA 10
hepatitis C SBA 10, EMQ 7
hepatosplenomegaly SBA 23,
SBA 104, SBA 108, EMQ 28
hepcidin SBA 88, SBA 91
hereditary haemorrhagic
telangiectasia SBA 11
hereditary xerocytosis SBA 115
herpes zoster vaccination
SBA 110
Heyde syndrome SBA 11
HIV/AIDS SBA 9, SBA 10,
SBA 117

Hodgkin lymphoma SBA 14,
SBA 53, EMQ 6, EMQ 9,
EMQ 25
nodular lymphocyte-
predominant (NLPHL) --9
horse antithymocyte globulin
SBA 62
human immunodeficiency virus
see HIV/AIDS
hydrops fetalis SBA 23
hydroxycarbamide SBA 103,
SBA 112
hyperbilirubinaemia SBA 35
hypercalcaemia SBA 67
hypercholesterolaemia SBA 7,
SBA 39
hyperdiploidy SBA 114
hyperhaemolysis EMQ 27
hypertension SBA 46
hypochromia SBA 23
hyponatraemia SBA 40
hypoparathyroidism SBA 33
hypotension SBA 12
hypothyroidism SBA 14
hypotransferrinaemia EMQ 22

ibrutinib SBA 76
idiopathic bile salt malabsorption
SBA 25
IgA anti-tissue transglutaminase
antibodies SBA 8
IgM myeloma EMQ 14
imatinib SBA 52, SBA 75
immune deficiency SBA 2
immune drug-induced microangiopathy EMQ 4
immunoglobulin, intravenous
EMQ 13
infliximab SBA 2

INR SBA 7, SBA 39, SBA 48,
   SBA 50, SBA 109
International Normalised Ratio
   see INR
intrahepatic cholestasis, sickle
   cell-related SBA 35
intrinsic factor antibodies
   SBA 32, SBA 100
inv(16)(p13.1q22) EMQ 28
involved field radiotherapy
   SBA 53, EMQ 9
irbesartan SBA 47
iron deficiency anaemia SBA 5,
   SBA 8, SBA 11, EMQ 8
iron-refractory SBA 88
iron overload SBA 33
irritable bowel syndrome SBA 8

JAK2 mutation SBA 43, SBA 54,
   SBA 58
jaundice EMQ 26
JC virus SBA 2
juvenile myelomonocytic
   leukaemia SBA 61, SBA 96

Katayama fever SBA 28

lactate dehydrogenase (LDH)
   SBA 29
Langerhans cell histiocytosis
   SBA 87
langerin SBA 87
large B-cell lymphoma SBA 117
lead poisoning SBA 6
leucoencephalopathy, progressive
   multifocal SBA 2
leucoerythroblastic SBA 34
leucopenia SBA 29
leukaemia

acute lymphoblastic SBA 14,
   SBA 81
acute myeloid SBA 13, SBA 31,
   SBA 83
acute myelomonocytic
   EMQ 28
acute promyelocytic SBA 77
chronic eosinophilic SBA 75
chronic lymphocytic SBA 1,
   SBA 76, SBA 110, EMQ 12
chronic myelogenous SBA 52,
   SBA 116
chronic myelomonocytic
   EMQ 28
hairy cell EMQ 12
juvenile myelomonocytic
   SBA 61, SBA 96
plasma cell SBA 12
T-cell prolymphocytic EMQ 1,
   EMQ 19
leukaemia cutis SBA 104
livedo reticularis SBA 21
liver disease SBA 50
low molecular weight heparin
   SBA 82
lung cancer SBA 48
lupus anticoagulant SBA 21,
   SBA 82
lymphadenopathy SBA 40,
   SBA 41, SBA 51, EMQ 12
lymphocytosis EMQ 12
lymphoma EMQ 7
angioimmunoblastic T-cell
   EMQ 1
B-cell SBA 92
B-cell, unclassifiable SBA 67
Burkitt SBA 41, SBA 79,
   SBA 85, EMQ 12, EMQ 24
diffuse large B-cell SBA 37

lymphoma (*continued*)
 extranodal marginal zone
   SBA 69
 extranodal NK/T-cell, nasal type
   EMQ 1
 follicular EMQ 24
 Hodgkin SBA 14, SBA 53,
   EMQ 6, EMQ 9, EMQ 25
 large B-cell SBA 117
 mantle cell SBA 2, EMQ 12
lymphoproliferative disorders
 acute lymphoblastic leukaemia
   SBA 14, SBA 81
 autoimmune lymphoproliferative syndrome SBA 63
 B-cell lymphoma SBA 67,
   SBA 92
 chronic lymphocytic leukaemia
   SBA 1, SBA 76, SBA 110,
   EMQ 12
 follicular lymphoma EMQ 24
 hairy cell leukaemia EMQ 12
 multiple myeloma SBA 114,
   SBA 119

magnetic resonance imaging
   (MRI) SBA 78
malaria SBA 29, EMQ 29
mantle cell lymphoma SBA 2,
   EMQ 12
May-Hegglin anomaly EMQ 5
megaloblastic anaemia SBA 16,
   SBA 18, SBA 22
meningococcal septicaemia
   SBA 27
methaemoglobinaemia
   SBA 106
methotrexate SBA 13, SBA 92
methylene blue SBA 106

microangiopathic haemolytic
   anaemia SBA 73, EMQ 29
microcytosis SBA 23,
   SBA 108
monoclonal gammopathy of
   undetermined significance
   (MGUS) EMQ 14
monocytosis SBA 45
MPL mutation SBA 58
multiple myeloma SBA 114,
   SBA 119
myalgia SBA 28
MYC gene SBA 85
mycophenolate mofetil SBA 2,
   SBA 113
Mycoplasma pneumoniae EMQ 29
mycosis fungoides EMQ 19
myelodysplastic syndrome
   SBA 90, EMQ 16
 hypoplastic SBA 70
myelofibrosis
 post-polycythaemia SBA 97
 primary SBA 34, SBA 60
myeloid sarcoma EMQ 19
myeloma, IgM EMQ 14
MYH9 EMQ 5, EMQ 17

natalizumab SBA 2
needle prick injuries SBA 10
neonate
 congenital heart disease
   SBA 105
 Down syndrome SBA 104
 exchange transfusion SBA 101
 Rh haemolytic disease SBA 101
neoplasms
 brain tumour SBA 92
 breast cancer SBA 14, SBA 34,
   SBA 71, SBA 85, SBA 116

lung cancer SBA 48
myeloid sarcoma EMQ 19
neural tube defects SBA 15
neurofibromatosis EMQ 10
neutropenia SBA 63
autoimmune EMQ 16
drug-induced EMQ 16
ethnic EMQ 16
neutrophilic leukaemoid reaction
SBA 119
neutrophils SBA 3, SBA 4,
SBA 5, SBA 12
dysplastic SBA 31
leucocytosis SBA 36
night sweats SBA 65

oedema SBA 7
oral anticoagulants SBA 46
osteoporosis SBA 113

pancytopenia SBA 62, EMQ 12,
EMQ 21
paracentesis SBA 90
parasitic infection SBA 28, EMQ
25
paroxysmal cold haemoglobinuria
EMQ 26
paroxysmal nocturnal
haemoglobinuria SBA 56
parvovirus B19 EMQ 27, EMQ 29
pathogen-inactivated fresh frozen
plasma EMQ 11
PDGFRA rearrangement EMQ 25
PDGFRB rearrangement
SBA 75
peripheral neuropathy SBA 102
pernicious anaemia SBA 100
petechiae SBA 86, EMQ 13
phlebotomy SBA 89

phytosterolaemia EMQ 30
plasma cell leukaemia SBA 12
plasma exchange SBA 73,
EMQ 23
plasmacytoma SBA 102
plasmapheresis SBA 80
Plasmodium falciparum EMQ 29
platelet count SBA 58
platelet transfusion EMQ 13
plegmasia caerulea dolens SBA 7
POEMS syndrome SBA 102,
EMQ 10, EMQ 14
poikilocytosis SBA 22, SBA 23,
SBA 108, EMQ 22
polychromasia SBA 6, SBA 17,
SBA 25
polyclonal B lymphocytosis
SBA 120
polycythaemia, cyanotic heart
disease SBA 105
polycythaemia vera SBA 43,
SBA 54, SBA 97, SBA 103,
SBA 112
polymyalgia rheumatica SBA 20
prednisolone SBA 37, SBA 40,
SBA 42, SBA 113
prednisone EMQ 6
pregnancy
β thalassaemia heterozygosity
SBA 99
Burkitt lymphoma SBA 85
coeliac disease SBA 15
haemoglobin O-Arab SBA 118
lupus anticoagulant SBA 82
thalassaemia SBA 95
priapism SBA 35
procarbazine EMQ 6
progressive multifocal leucoencephalopathy SBA 2

prothrombin complex SBA 48
prothrombin concentrate
EMQ 11
prothrombin time (PT) SBA 4,
SBA 21, SBA 25, SBA 27,
SBA 49, SBA 55
pseudohyperkalaemia SBA 115
pulmonary angiography SBA 44
pulmonary embolism SBA 44,
SBA 48, SBA 107, SBA 109
pure red cell aplasia SBA 18
purpura SBA 19
pyridoxine SBA 89
pyrimidine 5' nucleotidase
deficiency EMQ 30
pyropoikilocytosis, hereditary
EMQ 30

5q syndrome EMQ 18
quinine EMQ 4

R-CHOP regimen SBA 37,
SBA 40
rasburicase SBA 37, SBA 79
red cell distribution width (RDW)
SBA 6, SBA 100
red cells SBA 11
fragments SBA 22
nucleated SBA 6, SBA 17,
SBA 23
transfusion SBA 66
renal failure EMQ 12,
EMQ 27
renal transplantation SBA 92
reticulocytosis SBA 63
Rh haemolytic disease of newborn
SBA 101
rheumatoid arthritis SBA 5,
SBA 30

rheumatoid factor SBA 1
ring sideroblasts SBA 6, SBA 89,
EMQ 18
rituximab SBA 2, SBA 37,
SBA 40, SBA 68, SBA 110,
SBA 113, SBA 117, EMQ 9
rivaroxaban SBA 47
rosuvastatin SBA 47
rouleaux formation SBA 5,
SBA 119
RPS19 EMQ 17
ruxolitinib SBA 60, SBA 97,
SBA 112

schistosomiasis SBA 28,
EMQ 25
sepsis SBA 83
septic transfusion reaction
EMQ 3
septicaemia EMQ 29
Sézary syndrome SBA 51,
EMQ 19
Shwachman-Diamond syndrome
EMQ 21
sickle cell disease SBA 35,
SBA 59, EMQ 27
sideroblastic anaemia, congenital
EMQ 22
sinusoidal obstruction syndrome
SBA 13, SBA 90
sirolimus SBA 90
skin plaques SBA 64
smoking SBA 120
solvent-detergent-treated fresh
frozen plasma SBA 80,
EMQ 2
spherocytosis, hereditary
SBA 24
splenectomy SBA 12

splenic sequestration EMQ 27
splenomegaly SBA 34, SBA 40,
    SBA 41, SBA 52, SBA 60,
    SBA 120, EMQ 12
stomatocytosis, overhydrated
    hereditary EMQ 30
Streptococcus pneumonia SBA 12
syndrome of inappropriate
    secretion of antidiuretic
    hormone (SIADH) SBA 40
systemic lupus erythematosus
    (SLE) SBA 18, SBA 21
systemic mastocytosis SBA 45,
    EMQ 10

T-cell precursor lymphoblastic
    leukaemia/lymphoma
    EMQ 1
T-cell prolymphocytic leukaemia
    EMQ 1, EMQ 19
t(1;22)(p13;q13) EMQ 28
t(5;12)(q31-33;p12) EMQ 28
t(6;9)(p23;q34) EMQ 28
t(8;14)(q24;q32) EMQ 24
t(9;22)(q34;q1SBA 2) EMQ 24
t(11;14)(q13;q32) EMQ 24
t(12;21)(p13;q22) EMQ 24
t(14;18)(q32;q21) EMQ 24
t(15;17)(q22;q12) EMQ 28
tacrolimus SBA 13
target cells SBA 115
teardrop poikilocytes SBA 22,
    SBA 97
temporal arteritis SBA 42
thalassaemia
    α^+ thalassaemia EMQ 8
    α^0 thalassaemia SBA 98,
    EMQ 15, EMQ 20,
    EMQ 22

β thalassaemia SBA 23,
    SBA 99, SBA 118, EMQ 8,
    EMQ 15, EMQ 20
β^+ thalassaemia SBA 95
β^0 thalassaemia SBA 108
$\delta\beta$ thalassaemia SBA 108,
    EMQ 22
thalassaemia intermedia SBA 78
thalassaemia major SBA 33
thalassaemia trait SBA 43
therapy-related myeloid neoplasm
    SBA 71
thrombin time (TT) SBA 25,
    SBA 84
thrombocythaemia, essential
    SBA 34, SBA 54
thrombocytopenia SBA 16,
    SBA 29, SBA 36
    with absent radii EMQ 21
    alloimmune EMQ 5
    heparin-induced SBA 107
thrombocytosis SBA 116
thrombotic thrombocytopenic
    purpura (TTP) SBA 9,
    EMQ 4, EMQ 23
    hereditary EMQ 4
tissue plasminogen activator
    SBA 39
TMPRSS6 mutation SBA 88
tolvaptan SBA 40
total iron binding capacity SBA 5
toxic granulation SBA 12,
    SBA 119
tranexamic acid EMQ 2, EMQ 11
transfusion reactions
    acute haemolytic EMQ 3
    anaphylactic EMQ 3
    delayed haemolytic EMQ 26
    septic EMQ 3

transfusion-associated acute lung
    injury (TRALI) EMQ 3
transient abnormal myelopoiesis
    SBA 104
tryptase SBA 45
tumour lysis syndrome SBA 37,
    SBA 41, SBA 79
tyrosine kinase inhibitors
    SBA 76

vaccination
    herpes zoster SBA 110
    varicella-zoster SBA 26
varicella-zoster vaccination
    SBA 26
vasculitis SBA 20
venesection SBA 103
vinblastine SBA 14
vincristine SBA 37, SBA 40,
    EMQ 6
vitamin B_{12} deficiency SBA 22,
    SBA 94, EMQ 18

vitamin K SBA 48,
    SBA 107
malabsorption SBA 25
von Willebrand disease SBA 11,
    SBA 66, SBA 74
acquired SBA 55
von Willebrand factor SBA 66,
    SBA 80

warfarin SBA 7, SBA 39,
    SBA 46, SBA 48,
    SBA 109
warm autoimmune haemolytic
    anaemia SBA 113
weight loss SBA 20, SBA 65
Wells' score SBA 38
Wilms tumour SBA 55
Wilson's disease SBA 17
Wiskott-Aldrich syndrome
    EMQ 5

Zieve's syndrome SBA 17

Printed and bound by CPI Group (UK) Ltd, Croydon, CR0 4YY

10/06/2025

14686701-0001